The
Rehabilitation
Detectives

SOCIOLOGICAL OBSERVATIONS

Series Editor: **JOHN M. JOHNSON,** Arizona State University

"This new series seeks its inspiration primarily from its subject matter and the nature of its observational setting. It draws on all academic disciplines and a wide variety of theoretical and methodological perspectives. The series has a commitment to substantive problems and issues and favors research and analysis which seek to blend actual observations of human actions in daily life with broader theoretical, comparative, and historical perspectives. SOCIOLOGICAL OBSERVATIONS aims to use all of our available intellectual resources to better understand all facets of human experience and the nature of our society."

—John M. Johnson

The
Rehabilitation
Detectives

Doing Human Service Work

Paul C. Higgins

SAGE PUBLICATIONS
The Publishers of Professional Social Science
Beverly Hills   London   New Delhi

For information address:

SAGE Publications, Inc.
275 South Beverly Drive
Beverly Hills, California 90212

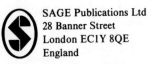

SAGE Publications India Pvt. Ltd.
M-32 Market
Greater Kailash I
New Delhi 110 048 India

SAGE Publications Ltd
28 Banner Street
London EC1Y 8QE
England

Printed in the United States of America

Library of Congress Cataloging in Publication Data

Main entry under title:

Higgins, Paul C.
    The rehabilitation detectives.

    (Sociological observation; v. 16)
    Bibliography: p.
    Includes index.
    1. Rehabilitation counselors. 2. Rehabilitation counselors—Case Studies. I. Title. II. Series: Sociological observations ; 16.
HD7255.5.H55   1985   362'.0425   85-1849
ISBN 0-8039-2450-X
ISBN 0-8039-2451-8 (pbk.)

FIRST PRINTING

Contents

*To my wife, Leigh, whose competence and caring
in teaching hearing-impaired children is what
human service work should be*

PREFACE
Detective Work

Gary L. Albrecht

University of Illinois at Chicago

The street is an office for both the social scientist and the human service worker. If we want to find out what people are doing and understand their behavior, we have to go take a look. If researchers and service providers are to touch those they serve or understand the people in their studies, they must "hang out" on the street. Managers of human service workers and dissertation directors, therefore, are happiest when their minions are out in the field, for the streets are where ideas are generated and hunches validated.

Paul Higgins uses the metaphor of the rehabilitation detective to take us vicariously into the world of vocational counselors and their clients. He challenges professionals who construct their work world through meetings and paper documents to revisit their primary work site, the street. Once we venture into the world of the vocational rehabilitation counselor, we discover that the nostrums of researchers and politicians often are not tenable. Human service workers and their clients frequently are intelligent, reasonable, and responsive, but they operate within the boundaries of a complex world where clear principles seldom pertain. Often, what appears rational to external observers makes no sense to the participants. Theirs is the world of trade-offs designed to reap rewards for and minimize risk to counselor and client. Paul Higgins takes us inside the operational dynamics of this social world.

Rehabilitation detectives are sleuths and managers trying to maintain a balance among multiple forces in the social service arena. These counselors are enjoined to make the system work and, simultaneously, to "look good." In fact, appearances are more important than reality. Given a public mandate, it is more important for service organizations and counselors to look good than actually to help the client. This does not release them, however, from their concomitant obligation to serve the public. For, while achievement of the public good requires that the culture and norms of the community be upheld by major institutions, counselors recognize at the same time that the good of the individual also should be protected. Negotiation and maintenance of this balance is a major component of the rehabilitation counselor's job.

The fundamental task of the counselor involves constructing, managing, and vindicating an appropriate social self for the client that will meet the test of the organization. A classic illustration of this activity is provided through the words of a functionally blind vocational counselor I interviewed some years ago in Detroit:

> One day about twelve years ago a teenage inner-city Black kid was brought to me. The mother and friends pleaded with me to accept this kid for services but I said, "Man, the kid is young, blind, isn't doing well in school. What job is he goin' to get. What are we goin' to train him for?" The kid spoke up, "I'm a musician. Listen to me. I want to play the piano and go to Hollywood." I can't see either and I had dreams I couldn't meet. This kid . . . he had a dream. I could feel it in my gut. He was goin' to make it. But, there was no way I could get him on the rolls according to the rules. My supervisor said "no dice" so I took the kid under my wing and massaged a few of the rules. He got piano and music lessons. Man, what a thrill when Stevie Wonder paid my way to Hollywood years later to watch him get an Emmy. We showed 'em. I was right and then they wanted to take credit for it, but Stevie and I knew the story.

This vocational counselor exulted in the success of his risk-taking behavior, which resulted in a triumph for the client, the counselor, and the agency. Everyone won. Yet, even by his own admission, such success stories are moderated by the risky human investments that pay meager dividends. The work life of a rehabilitation counselor involves a continual calculus of risk in making allocational decisions. In the Stevie Wonder case, the counselor was faced with a difficult set of facts but decided to bend some rules based on a "gut reaction" to the individual and a personal knowledge of visual impairment. The counselor's street experience and insider's view of the system accounted for his good decision.

The exercise of complex decision models used in determining client eligibility is difficult because often it is disrupted by unpredictable events: The state runs out of money for services before the end of the fiscal year, the demand for services increases with unemployment, or there are few jobs in which to place clients. Therefore, to be successful the counselor needs to know how to make the case. Stevie Wonder's counselor is not unique. Proficient human service workers are able to weigh the advantages of receiving services against the disadvantages of being labeled. They are able to make complex decisions about the best use of resources in specific cases, keeping in mind the dual goals of looking good while helping those in need. Since the human service delivery business is characterized both by self-serving interests and *pro bono* ideologies and actions, sensitive and sophisticated analyses are needed. Paul Higgins provides us with a firsthand description and analysis of this complex social world. His work stands in the best tradition of sociological fieldwork. May it stimulate others to move their offices out into the street.

Acknowledgments

Social research is always a collective enterprise. The finished product may be typed and retyped or nowadays entered on a word processor by others. Colleagues read and comment upon rough drafts. Universities provide institutional support. Previous research and writing of others stimulate one's own work. And, of course, there are the social actors who are the focus of the investigation.

Without the cooperation of the rehabilitation counselors and the other professionals within the rehabilitation agency in which my research was conducted, this book would not have been possible. To let an outsider come in and observe showed courage and confidence. I wish that I could publicly identify the rehabilitation professionals, but to do so would destroy their anonymity, which I promised to maintain.

Jaber F. Gubrium, John M. Johnson, and Robert L. Stewart read previous drafts of this book and provided many useful suggestions.

I appreciate the support of my department of sociology. That support enabled many people, in particular Mrs. Jo Ann Hess, to transcribe tape recordings of my observations and to type and retype drafts of this book.

To all those who helped in this collective enterprise, thanks.

INTRODUCTION

This is kind of a tricky case.

So you know you have to rely on what they tell you to a great extent, too, but then you also have to, you know, dig around and get some other information as well.

So what are you saying I do with this one? / You are going to have to look at it and make your decision. Do you feel like it's a case? / I do.

Sounds like a good case.

The above remarks are not those of law enforcement detectives discussing criminal cases and investigations. They are the remarks of another kind of detective: vocational rehabilitation counselors. They are the rehabilitation detectives. What follows is a "story" of the work of rehabilitation counselors and more generally of human service professionals.

SOCIOLOGICAL FRAMEWORKS

One of the promises, as well as one of the tasks, of the social sciences is to develop frameworks through which the social world can be understood. Whether we call those frameworks "theoretical perspectives," "schemes," "sensitizing concepts" (Blumer, 1969), or "stories" (Davis, 1974), they enable us to give coherence to an otherwise odd assortment of observations. Through these frameworks we develop a basic understanding of the social world. They remain with us, to be used again and again, long after the facts and figures have been forgotten.

For example, several years ago I wrote *Outsiders in a Hearing World,* a sociological analysis of the lives of people who are deaf. I saw deaf people as outsiders in two related ways. First, they live within a world of sounds, a world in which being able to hear (and speak) is not only important, but also taken for granted. Yet deaf people are not fully part of that world. In this obvious sense they are outsiders in a hearing world. Second, and more significant, deaf people are outsiders in a world largely created and controlled by those who hear. Based on historically changing assumptions about deafness and deaf people, the hearing have decided what educational, occupational, and other opportunities are to be made available to deaf people. Thus deaf people "live within a world which is not of their own making, but one which they must continually confront" (Higgins, 1980: 22). From this perspective, I tried to understand and clarify deaf people's lives. Of course, the specifics of deaf people's lives are important. However, the concept of "outsiders" helps us to make sense of those specifics, sensitizes us to new areas of inquiry, and will be with us long after the specifics are forgotten.

If developed well, these frameworks enable us to see the social world in ways we had not seen it before. As Joseph Gusfield (1976: 32) notes:

> It is the capacity to recognize the context of unexamined assumptions and accepted concepts that is among the most valuable contributions through which social science enables human beings to transcend the conventional and create new approaches and policies.

Thus the metaphor of "detective" may enable us to transcend the conventional and commonsense view of rehabilitation counselors.

These frameworks do more than help us make sense of our observations. They suggest to us possibilities, connections within the social world that we have yet to investigate. They help us see similarities among social phenomena where only differences were initially noted; and, they help us see differences where only similarities were thought to exist. For example, not only are deaf people outsiders in a hearing world, but black Americans are outsiders in a white world and gays are outsiders in a straight world. The concept of "outsiders" helps us to notice significant similarities among people who otherwise are thought to be quite different. Conversely, while two elderly adults, one deaf due to aging and the other deaf from birth, may have similar hearing losses, their lives are likely to be worlds apart. The first is a hearing person who happens to have had a hearing loss. The second is a deaf person, an outsider in a hearing world.

The "detective" metaphor may be similarly instructive. Vocational rehabilitation counselors, social service workers, mental health professionals, parole agents, and other human service professionals may have a great deal in common in addition to providing services to people. They may in fact have a great deal in common with detectives. With increased emphasis on bureaucracies in the human services, where clients are processed on a mass level (Weatherley, 1979: 145), rehabilitation counselors and other human service professionals increasingly find themselves handling cases and not simply serving people. Conversely, *from this viewpoint,* there may be relatively fewer ties that bind rehabilitation counselors to clinical psychologists, therapists, ministers, and others who guide and counsel.

As any good storyteller knows, stories that contain many plots may become confusing. The same is true for sociological frameworks. While they enable us to understand a variety of observations, they cannot help us organize all the observations we have made. Frameworks can encompass only so much material. They help give meaning to what we include, but they also necessitate that we exclude. We cannot tell everything in one story, within one framework. What we exclude might be appropriately understood within other frameworks, left for other storytellers to tell.

Therefore, just as *Outsiders in a Hearing World* was *one* sociological story of the lives of deaf people and not the *only* possible story, so it is with this work. It is just one look at vocational rehabilitation counselors and human service professionals through a particular framework. It does not tell everything one might want to know about rehabilitation counselors. It does not even tell all I have learned about rehabilitation counselors. Other stories could and must be told.

While the story told here is based primarily on observations of one area office of one state vocational rehabilitation agency, its scope is not limited to that one office or state agency, or even to rehabilitation counselors. Though the specifics of the story are likely to vary as one moves further from the area office described—to other area offices, to other state vocational rehabilitation agencies, to other human service agencies—the framework may prove useful for understanding what human service professionals do in a large variety of settings. Even the specifics may often be similar because the human service professionals are doing their work under similar circumstances. Thus a story about rehabilitation detectives becomes more generally a story about human service detectives.

What a story says to a reader depends, to a great extent, on what the reader brings to the story. Different readers will come away with different understandings because their purposes in reading the story and the experiences they bring to it will differ markedly. Regardless, if social scientists use different frameworks in order to tell different stories about the "same" social world, then surely different readers of the "same" story can come away with different understandings.

This volume is aimed at several different audiences: social scientists and students interested in disability and organizations that serve those with disabilities, those interested more broadly in human service organizations, professionals in rehabilitation and in human services, and concerned citizens. Even those interested in detective work, whether it concerns crime or not, may find this story useful. However, what is novel and instructive to one group of readers may be well known to another. Thus a difficult balancing act is attempted between stating what is obvious to some and taking too much for granted with others.

ORDINARY PEOPLE

The following chapters describe and analyze how ordinary people do their jobs as rehabilitation detectives, as vocational rehabilitation counselors and, more generally, as human service professionals. In using the term "ordinary people," I do not mean to denigrate or belittle vocational rehabilitation counselors, certainly not those who allowed me to be a part of their work world. Instead, I use the term to emphasize that rehabilitation counselors and human service professionals are just like you and me. We are made of the same stuff. Ordinary people can be caring and despairing, considerate and rude, concerned and indifferent. They can go out of their way to help some, and they can deprecate those who do not lift a finger to help themselves. They can work long past quitting time, and they can watch the clock on Friday afternoon. Ordinary people are human; neither saints nor sinners, yet at times a bit of both. So it is with rehabilitation detectives.

Too often we mystify other people. We caricature them and, in doing so, we set them apart from ourselves. Teachers of children with disabilities have enormous patience; artists are slightly odd; librarians are repressed; and police officers are authoritarian. Depending on one's point of view, human service professionals are compassionate, cold (bureaucratic), or indifferent, or have some other attribute that signifies they are somehow different from us. This mystical difference is then used to explain what these folks do, whether they be teachers, artists, librarians, police officers, or human service professionals. In overlooking the "ordinariness" that we share, we jump too quickly to "person-pointing" (and often faulting) in order to understand what people do (see McKinlay, 1978: 31-32).

Within social scientists' concerns about human service organizations, one focus is on the "unsanctioned behavior of policemen, social workers, medical personnel, assistant district attorneys, employment office officials, and countless other low-level bureaucrats" (Prottas, 1979: 163). While that unsanctioned behavior may be seen as a response to the organizational and social circumstances under which the "low-level bureaucrats" work, the bottom line is that often such bureaucrats and their behavior need to be "shaped up" so human services can be provided more equitably.[1] No doubt, instances abound in which that is true. But to say only that is merely to point one's finger at human service providers, who with the intentions and skills of ordinary people are doing their work in ways others find unacceptable. We may as well point the finger at all of us, for we are all fallible.

Rather than pointing a finger, I will try to describe and explain how rehabilitation counselors do their work within an organizational and social context. From the descriptions of the counselor's behaviors, some may infer laudable or disagreeable qualities about those people, *that would be a mistake.* To psychologize what rehabilitation counselors do, whether we deem it praiseworthy or blameworthy, overlooks the social circumstances in which they do what they do. Certainly, counselors (and ordinary people) vary on attributes we admire or dislike. But to focus primarily on those attributes encourages us needlessly to make invidious distinctions, and often misleads us to think that "getting better people" is *the* way to make improvements (see Lipsky, 1980: xv).

PLAN OF THE BOOK

In the following chapters I describe and analyze what vocational rehabilitation counselors do. To do so, I use the metaphor of detective work. Chapter 1 establishes that framework, which is then used in subsequent chapters. However, rehabilitation counselors are not the only human service detectives. Social service and mental health caseworkers, parole agents, child welfare workers, drug abuse counselors, and other human service professionals are detectives, too. Therefore, I draw on information about other human service professionals in order to tell a broader story.

Rehabilitation counselors do their work within an organization. The philosophy, policies, procedures, and people that constitute the organization provide the setting within which rehabilitation detective work is accomplished. What counselors do can be understood only within that organization, and what they do constitutes a significant part of the organization. Chapter 2 describes that setting.

In order to serve people who are vocationally handicapped due to disabilities, rehabilitation counselors must establish their eligibility for services. They must make a case for the client. Chapter 3 explores how rehabilitation counselors work cases in order to make a case for serving individuals with disabilities.

Once eligibility has been established, rehabilitation counselors seek to serve clients to enable them to remain or become successfully employed. However, cases do not always end successfully. Chapter 4 describes how rehabilitation detectives conclude cases.

Rehabilitation counselors work with many individuals simultaneously. At any given time, the individuals and their cases are at various stages in the rehabilitation process: Some are referrals, others are applicants whose eligibility is being investigated, and still others are clients who are being served in order to conclude their cases satisfactorily. Rehabilitation detectives cannot, and do not, solve one case before going on to the next. Instead, as Chapter 5 explains, counselors manage their caseloads. And in doing so, their concerns transcend the management of any individual case.

Specialization is important within both detective work and human service work. Much of detective work is done in details: the juvenile detail, burglary detail, or major crimes detail. While the basic nature of detective work is found in the various details, the details of a particular case may vary. So it is with the work of rehabilitation counselors. Many do rehabilitation work within specialty caseloads, where the specifics of the work vary. Chapter 6 examines four specialty caseloads in rehabilitation work.

Concern continues, perhaps even grows, regarding how well justice is served by detectives (and the criminal justice system of which they are a part) as well as how just (and efficient, effective, and so forth) is the service of rehabilitation counselors and other human service professionals and the agencies of which they are a part. Human service work is increasingly recognized as problematic. If service is not just, then why, and what can be done? In concluding this investigation, I address these two questions.

This story was based on my investigation of rehabilitation counselors. The Research Appendix explains my work as a sociological detective (Sanders, 1976). Of course, no crime had been committed. Rather, the problem was to make sense of what I was observing about rehabilitation counselors. As the jury, the readers can decide whether or not this case was successfully solved.

In part, my case rests on quotes from counselors and other rehabilitation professionals. Some of those quotes do not appear in grammatically correct form. This is no reflection on the competence of the rehabilitation detectives. We all speak and write ungrammatically at times. I tried not to modify significantly how these rehabilitation counselors wrote or talked.

Throughout this book I have tried to maintain the anonymity of those who shared their world with me. My concern is not that social scientists or students interested in disability, vocational rehabilitation, or human service work will recognize these detectives. They will not.

Instead, without anonymity, others in the vocational rehabilitation field—from the national level to the area office—would recognize these people. Therefore, no names appear. Information that would have identified specific people was generally deleted, although this was not always possible. For example, if only one rehabilitation counselor primarily handles clients with a certain disability, then to discuss working with such clients necessarily identifies the counselor, at least to fellow counselors. If a few counselors handle certain kinds of cases, then to discuss the working of those cases necessarily identifies a limited group of counselors, though not a specific counselor. Unproductive, even destructive, guessing games may ensue. Where that was a potential problem, I checked with the individuals involved. However, it is neither possible nor desirable to bowdlerize a sociological investigation such as this one. Nevertheless, detectives, whether they be of the law enforcement, human services, or sociological kind, often face difficult ethical decisions such as this in their work (Warren, 1980).

NOTE

1. The attitude toward "low-level bureaucrats" may at times be derisive or condescending:

> This is a story about magicians. But it is not a story about old crones in secluded hovels turning princes into frogs. It is about modern, mundane magicians, with powers more relevant to urban crisis than to sleeping princesses. Times have changed for magicians as for everyone else. The outputs of vast pharmaceutical laboratories can change princes into frogs (or anything else) far more easily and quickly than can even the most skilled old crone. What is called for in modern magic is mass marketing—the capacity to change a great number of citizens into a limited number of creatures economically and efficiently. For such magic 9 a.m. to 5 p.m. is a more propitious time than the full of the moon, and printed forms conjure better than bat-wings and are more readily available. These modern magicians are organization men and women. They work for welfare departments, police departments, hospitals, housing authorities, courts, and so forth, and if they can't change a citizen into a frog they can certainly do a goat and will generally try for a sheep. These practitioners of modern magic are frequently called bureaucrats—street-level bureaucrats (but who knows what Merlin was called behind his back). Their occult task is to turn ordinary citizens into "clients" (or "suspects," "patients," or any other trade name for client). This is a study of how they ply their trade [Prottas, 1979: 1].

1

THE REHABILITATION DETECTIVES

The detective's task is to solve crimes. The vocational rehabilitation counselor's task is to enable individuals with vocationally handicapping impairments to remain or to become successfully employed. The work of detectives and rehabilitation counselors could not be more different. Not so! One of the following quotes concerns detective work and one concerns the work of rehabilitation counselors:

> . . . and you start from there, and everything that you can compile from there will point to one direction, and if it doesn't you're out to lunch . . . and you have to start looking, you gotta find a point in which to go.

> * * *

> So that, you know, just little things like that sometimes will tell the tale on it. On the other day, he said he was working such and such a place and gave us a name and number. We can't find that person and the address he's given us is a vacant lot. So we tell him we have to have something better than that.

The first is a detective discussing a "wait-and-see" approach in order to decide whether something is evidence or a lead (Sanders, 1977: 24). The second is a rehabilitation counselor remarking on some of the problems encountered in verifying a client's employment.

While the object of rehabilitation counseling is not to solve crimes, as a metaphor, detective work can help us understand the work of rehabilitation counselors. Detective work sensitizes us to the active, investigative, case-solving and case-managing nature of rehabilitation work. While there are some striking similarities in how detectives and rehabilitation counselors actually do their work, those similarities should not be overstated. Detective work is used here as metaphor, not as description. A brief comparison of detective work and rehabilitation counseling follows.

DETECTIVE WORK[1]

As everyone knows, detectives try to solve crimes. Yet what is it that detectives do when they try to solve crimes? They "gather, organize, and use information about social behavior" (Sanders, 1977: 12). From a large variety of information about a possible crime, they try to make sense of what has happened and what may happen. Like a jigsaw puzzle master, the detective attempts to put a disparate collection of bits and pieces into a coherent whole. However, unlike those who do puzzles, the detective

> at the outset of a case has numerous pieces but does not know which pieces fit which puzzle or indeed, whether any of them belong in any puzzle at all [Sanders, 1977: 25].

Detectives, unlike puzzle-doers, do not know what the solution should be. They must complete the puzzle without knowing how the finished picture looks. Unlike puzzle-doers, who have all the pieces in front of them, detectives must also decide what actions and objects are part of the crime puzzle. As they develop a better idea of what happened, it becomes easier for them to decide which events and objects are part of the puzzle. In retrospect they may realize that seemingly insignificant, overlooked, or misidentified events and objects are important parts of the puzzle. To solve crimes, detectives must create a sense of order out of what is often disorderly and puzzling.

In solving crimes, detectives do not just ask for the facts. In fact, what is a significant fact—evidence or a lead—may not be realized until much later in the working of a case. Instead, detectives are guided by "assumptions about the nature of crime and criminals" (Sanders, 1977: 99). Based on these assumptions, detectives are able to work a case—to gather, organize, and use information in making sense out of what happened. For example, detectives are guided by the assumption that the offender and the victim often know one another in homicide cases. Therefore, detectives are likely to question relatives, friends, and acquaintances first. Without such an assumption, detectives would not know where to begin. These assumptions have an impact on all phases of detective work. They are brought to the job when one becomes a detective and develop out of experiences while one is a detective.

To solve crimes, detectives "work cases." In working a case, they attempt to establish a case, identify a suspect, locate the suspect, "cop the suspect," and then dispose of the case. While not all detective investigations follow this sequence, a "typical" one does (Sanders, 1977: 79).

When establishing a case, detectives seek to decide whether a reported incident is an instance of a specific crime. For example, is the report of an attempted murder to be viewed as that kind of crime, or is it more appropriately seen as a "glorified domestic"—a squabble between spouses (Sanders, 1977: 84)? Or is the report of a crime to be seen as any kind of crime at all? Phony reports, mistakes and misinterpretations are often made by citizens when notifying police of crimes.

Once established, many cases are disposed of immediately because they are seen as insignificant—not worthy of investigation—and/or as having few or no leads. If further investigations are made, then detectives attempt to identify the offender. Victims and witnesses are interviewed and physical evidence is analyzed. Once a suspect is positively identified, locating that suspect is typically easy. With a name in hand, detectives know where to look and with whom to talk in order to locate the suspect: schools, previous criminal records, the department of motor vehicles, family, friends, and so forth. In other cases, a stakeout may be used to locate suspects who are known through their MO (their *modus operandi*) but who are unnamed. After the arrest, detectives attempt to get the suspect to "cop out," to admit guilt, often by presenting irrefutable evidence. However, at times suspects may present irrefutable evidence of their innocence, thus re-creating for detectives the task of identifying a suspect.

When cases are cleared, detectives feel that they have successfully done their job. As far as detectives are concerned, a case is cleared when they have decided that the case has been solved and the suspect has been identified and, where appropriate, is in custody. A suspect in a minor offense who is now in another state will not likely be brought back. Suspects who get off on "technicalities" do not change detectives' views of solved cases. Some suspects may be warned rather than brought into custody. Others, of course, go to court. In all these instances detectives feel they have done their job—solving crimes.

Detectives solve crimes within an organization, which has an important impact on their work. Policies, paperwork, and fellow professional "crime fighters" are both resources for and obstacles to detectives in doing their job. And in doing their job, detectives face not only the task of solving individual crimes, but also that of handling many crimes at the same time. "Stats"—arrest and clearance-rate statistics—are often, though not always, important to how detectives do their job (Skolnick, 1966: 167-181; Sanders, 1977: 82-83; Waegel, 1981). They are an indication of the department's and the detective's work performances. Yet the detectives' performances—doing their job—exist only within that complex social arrangement known as a police department. And the police department, as well as the larger criminal justice system, exists within an often contradictory and conflictual society.

REHABILITATION COUNSELING

Vocational rehabilitation counselors do not seem to have anything in common with detectives. Rehabilitation counselors face the task of enabling individuals with physical or mental impairments that constitute substantial handicaps to employment to remain or become successfully employed. In responding to this task, counselors engage in many activities, such as arranging medical and vocational evaluations, developing a plan of services, counseling clients, exploring job possibilities with employers, and developing referral sources.[2] True, these and other activities have nothing to do with solving crimes. But rehabilitation counselors' task has a great deal to do with gathering, organizing, and using information in order to manage people's behaviors. They too try to make sense out of what has happened and is happening—with their clients instead of with possible crimes. They too try to put together a collection of bits and pieces of information into a coherent role—a coherent whole concerning their clients' impairments, vocational handicaps, and potential courses of action. Like detectives, rehabilitation counselors must create order out of what is often problematic and disorderly. Their task, however, is to solve rehabilitation puzzles, not crime puzzles. Consequently, how they do so may differ from how detectives solve their puzzles.

To rehabilitate individuals, counselors work cases. By using the term "case," I do not mean to imply that counselors see their clients as objects, though at times they may talk that way (Manus, 1975). The term "case" appears often in rehabilitation counseling: case folder, case development staffing, opening/closing cases, caseload, and so on. But then detectives may talk very casually at times about crime, yet still be very much concerned with and aware of the human tragedy of crime (Sanders, 1980). Feelings and emotions are an important feature of detective work, both rehabilitation detective work and the one more readily recognized, even if at times the manner in which detectives talk masks that importance.

In working cases, counselors attempt to identify potential clients, establish their eligibility, and develop and enact plans of services. If they are successful, then vocationally handicapped individuals will remain or become successfully employed. In particular, counselors "follow" a "series of precise and logical steps" that make up the vocational rehabilitation process (Leary and Tseng, 1974: 9). The process can be depicted as a sequence of status codes that reflects the activities of counselors, clients, and others involved in the process, as well as the progress of clients through the process (Bitter, 1979).

The Rehabilitation Process

Briefly, the rehabilitation process begins with individuals referred to the vocational rehabilitation program (status 00). Some referrals apply for services (02). Others do not and their cases are closed (08). Of those who apply, some are certified as eligible (10) after having been evaluated medically, vocationally, and, where appropriate, psychologically, educationally, and socially. Others are found ineligible and their cases too are closed (08). For some, an intensive evaluation, up to eighteen months long, may be used in order to determine eligibility (06). Once eligibiity has been determined, a rehabilitation plan based on the previous evaluation is developed by the counselors and clients (12). Due to a variety of reasons, such as a move out of state, inability to locate, or refusal of services, a small percentage of clients who are eligible for services, or for whom a rehabilitation plan has been developed without services having been initiated, are closed unsuccessfully (30). Typically, at least some services will be provided after plans have been developed.

A variety of services may be provided to clients. Counseling and guidance (14); restoration service such as medical or psychiatric treatment, surgery, hearing aids, and artificial limbs (16); and training, which may include personal, social, and work adjustment training, technical or trade schools, and college (18) are available where needed. Once services are successfully completed (20), then employment is secured (22) and maintained for a minimum of sixty days, until the client's cases are closed and the clients deemed successfully rehabilitated (26). Once services have been initiated, progress may be interrupted (24) due to a variety of reasons, such as clients' illnesses or counselors' inability to locate the clients. If services have been initiated, but successful employment is not obtained or, if obtained, significant services were not provided, then the cases will be closed as unsuccessful (28). For those clients whose cases are closed successfully, post-employment services are available to help the clients maintain employment (32) (Bitter, 1979: 38-40).

Within the detective metaphor, the rehabilitation process can be understood broadly in a different way. The process provides the rehabilitation detectives the formal framework for working cases in order to solve them successfully. Rehabilitation detectives must develop and maintain referral sources (informants), who bring to their attention possible cases to be worked (00). The detectives will not have personal contact with all of those possible cases, and for many of those they do, they will promptly screen them out as unsuitable without taking an application on them. Hence many individuals who could be recorded formally as having been involved in (the earliest stage of) the rehabilitation process are not. Likewise, not all complaints received by law enforcement agencies are recorded, whether or not they later might have been shown to be unfounded (that is, determined not to have been a crime) (McCleary et al., 1982).

If the rehabilitation detectives decide to pursue the possible cases, then they will take applications (02) and, through additional investigation, attempt to make a case that the applicants are eligible (10), that they have physical or mental impairments that create substantial handicaps to employment, and that rehabilitation services may reasonably be expected to enable the individuals to remain or become employed (Bitter, 1979). By questioning potential clients and sometimes individuals knowledgeable about them, arranging for medical, psychological, vocational, and other kinds of evaluations, obtaining records from other agencies, and discussing the cases with consultants, counselors may gather a wide variety of information. Information about the potential clients' impairments, functional limitations, capabilities, interests, and needed services may then be used to make a case for the potential clients. For example, individuals who complain of vision problems and dizziness may or may not have one or more impairments that qualify them for services. They may merely have an easily correctible vision impairment that would not qualify them for services. Or they may be suffering from diabetic retinopathy with attendant adjustment problems, which becomes the basis for their eligibility. However, counselors must make the case for eligibility. Clients are neither eligible nor ineligible. Instead, counselors make them eligible or ineligible. I do not mean this in any sleight-of-hand sense. Rather, just as detectives must decide as a result of their investigative activities whether an incident is a crime or not and if so, what kind of crime, so must rehabilitation counselors decide after their investigations if a potential client is eligible or not. Making a case becomes noticeable in difficult or problematic cases, but it is equally important, if also noticed less easily, in routine cases. This will become more clear later.

At times the cases may be particularly difficult, and intensive investigation with the assistance of other personnel (that is, rehabilitation personnel) is needed (06). Many potential cases (02) are closed early (08) because a case clearly cannot be made for the applicants. Either the applicants did not cooperate in some way or the rehabilitation detectives did not uncover suitable evidence in order to make a case for the applicants. Once a case has been established (10), then a plan of services is developed and justified (12). Cases in which clients become uncooperative, move, refuse further assistance, and the like before services are initiated may also be closed (30). When services are provided (14, 16, 18), the detectives attempt to manage the cases so that the services are completed (20), employment is secured (22), and the cases are successfully closed (26). However, setbacks may lead to interrupted (24) or even unsuccessful cases (28). Thus the rehabilitation process provides the framework within which the rehabilitation detectives do their work. However, it neither provides a detailed prescription for what they should do nor a description of what they actually do. The following chapters give a more detailed account of the work done by rehabilitation detectives.

Like detectives, rehabilitation counselors are guided by assumptions, assumptions about the nature of disabilities, vocational handicaps, and those who are limited by them as well as those who are not. For example, counselors assume that school-age clients will be likely to change their vocational interests, and that the jobs they secure may not be the jobs that had originally been planned. Therefore, they know amendments to the plans are likely to be needed. Or counselors assume the problems presented by those seeking services may not be the only problems being suffered. Therefore, they do not necessarily confine their investigations to the initial, presented problems. Rehabilitation counselors bring these assumptions to their tasks as well as develop them in the course of their work.

Like detective work, the work of rehabilitation counselors takes place in an organizational setting. Policies, procedures, paperwork, fellow professionals, and community agencies are both resources and obstacles in doing one's job. And, of course, there are the people who seek the services of the agency, typically many people. Consequently, like detectives, rehabilitation counselors handle many cases at the same time. To the people whose cases they handle, counselors are, to a great degree, the agency. Yet, the rehabilitation agency, like the criminal justice system, exists in an often contradictory and conflictual society, one that both shuns those with disabilities as well as extends a helping hand.

People-Processing and People-Changing

Both detectives and rehabilitation counselors solve cases. However, detectives do so in order to catch criminals while counselors do so in order to serve clients. Consequently, how detectives and rehabilitation counselors solve cases is likely to differ. An important though relative difference between detective work and rehabilitation counseling concerns the distinction between people-processing and people-changing. Human service organizations, such as public schools, hospitals, police departments, welfare agencies, and vocational rehabilitation departments, are engaged in one or both of two broad functions: *people-processing* and *people-changing* (Hasenfeld and English, 1974). A diagnostic clinic, a juvenile court, or an employment office primarily processes people. Each attempts to identify and assess a person's "attributes, social situation and public identity" (Hasenfeld, 1972: 257). The assessment of the client may then lead to changes through self-reactions and/or the reactions of others. For example, a juvenile court processes a youth suspected of delinquency that may lead to the youth's being committed to a state training facility where services to change the youth are provided. Other human service organizations attempt to change people. A speech and hearing clinic, a welfare agency, and a mental health facility attempt to change their clients through the "application of various modification and treatment technologies" (Hasenfeld and English, 1974: 5). They are providing people-changing services. However, these services are dependent upon the previous processing. For example, medical care is dependent upon the particular "sick" status that is conferred upon the patient (Hasenfeld, 1972).

Some human service organizations perform both functions, people-processing and people-changing. Hospitals diagnose (that is, they process) as well as provide treatment (that is, they change the patient). Vocational rehabilitation departments in general and rehabilitation counselors in particular provide both services. Detective work, as predominantly characterized, primarily involves people-processing, though the criminal justice system of which detectives are a part processes and changes people.[3]

While vocational rehabilitation departments provide people-changing services, many of these services are not provided by rehabilitation counselors. Some are provided through agencies and by professionals in the community such as hospitals, drug clinics, technical schools, doctors, and psychologists. Other services may be provided by other rehabilitation professionals within the agency such as workshop staff who provide personal, social, and work adjustment training— training to improve money and time skills, hygiene, grooming, and other personal, social and work skills, which might include learning to become dependable and punctual, learning production speed on a task, and developing the ability to take supervision. To understand the provisions of these services would require other investigations. Likewise, to understand the work of various "evidence experts" in crime labs, work that does have a bearing on detectives' activities, might also require other investigations.

Among the services rehabilitation counselors provide directly is counseling and guidance, also known as "C and G." One would expect counselors to counsel and guide, and rehabilitation counselors indeed do.[4] As I explain later, if they cannot show the need for C and G, then they do not have a case, and if they have not provided any meaningful C and G to clients, then they will not have a successful case. However, counseling and guidance as a distinct activity was not a focus of my investigation and is not a focus of this story. By not focusing on it, I do not mean to suggest that it is not important. I would (partially) agree with counselors who "swear by it," though research is more equivocal. Counseling and guidance exists as talk. When rehabilitation counselors counsel and guide they talk, but they also talk without counseling and guiding. A detailed analysis of "doing counseling and guiding" would certainly be useful. I have not attempted such a study though much of what I discuss under various features of rehabilitation detective work would likely be discussed under "doing counseling and guidance."[5]

During the provision of services, a great deal of detective work takes place. In order to conclude cases that have been successfully made, clients' involvement in services must be maintained, jobs located, employment for the clients secured, successful performance on the jobs maintained for a minimum length of time, and all of this must be documented. The second quote at the beginning of this chapter is one small indication of the detective work needed at this stage of the rehabilitation process.

While the work of vocational rehabilitation counselors may be understood usefully within the metaphor of detective work, so may the work of other human service professionals. Rehabilitation counselors are not alone in working, making, and concluding cases. Wherever people's eligibility as clients for an agency's services must be established, plans of services developed and enacted, and the cases brought to a conclusion, human service detectives are at work. In public welfare agencies, mental health clinics, drug abuse centers, and other "street-level bureaucracies," low-level but often professional employees are the intermediaries between their agencies and the citizens to be served (Lipsky, 1980). One of their responsibilities is the "transformation of citizens into clients," which is "actualized via the decision to categorize a client in one way or another" (Prottas, 1979: 4). The transformation involves detective work: gathering, organizing, and using information to solve cases. Just as detectives decide which crimes to investigate among the many brought to their attention, so does the professional staff of community mental health centers decide whom to serve among potential clients (Emerson and Pollner, 1978; Lang, 1981; Peyrot, 1982). Or, a "modern parole agency is expected not only to supervise but also to diagnose, classify, and certify parolees" (McCleary, 1978: 20). To do so requires investigative work. Caseworkers within one state's social services department were formerly even called "investigators" (Gell, 1969; see also Zimmerman, 1966). Therefore, I draw on materials concerning other human service professionals in order to broaden our understanding of rehabilitation detectives, and in understanding the work of rehabilitation detectives, we deepen our knowledge of human service work.

VOCATIONAL REHABILITATION

The goal of rehabilitation is to restore or to enable individuals who have become impaired in some way to become as self-sufficient as possible (Bitter, 1979). Hospitals, mental health facilities, drug clinics, prisons, therapists, doctors, counselors, and many other facilities and professionals are involved in providing rehabilitation services. While all attempt to restore, the specific goals of the various agencies and professionals may differ. Hospitals and medical personnel are concerned primarily with physiological functioning; mental health facilities and professionals with psychological functioning; and correctional facilities and staff with social behavior and attitudes. Vocational rehabilitation agencies are concerned with employablity and employment. What follows is a very brief description of the history and philosophy of public vocational rehabilitation in America.[6]

The public vocational rehabilitation program began with the Vocational Rehabilitation Act of 1920, though federal, state, and private services had been provided before that time. The original act was quite modest in scope and in its initial implementation. As interpreted, the original act of 1920

> provided funds only for vocational guidance, training, occupational adjustment, prostheses, and placement services. Rehabilitation services were to be for the physically disabled and were to be vocational in nature. They could not include physical restoration or socially oriented rehabilitation [Bitter, 1979: 16].

The minimum age for eligibility was taken to be the minimum age of legal employability within the state. Homemaking was seen as a legitimate occupation. In anticipation of the federal act, a few states had previously passed enabling legislation in order to take advantage of the federal funds that were available on a 50/50 matching basis. Many other states quickly passed such legislation so that within 18 months, 34 states had begun to develop vocational rehabilitation programs (Lassiter, 1972).

The early thrust of state vocational rehabilitation agencies was to serve indigent people with orthopedic disabilities. Some services, such as counseling and guidance, were available to the nonpoor and limited services were available to those who were physically handicapped, but not orthopedically so (Lassiter, 1972). In 1920 federal appropriation to the states was $500,000 (Obermann, 1965: 225), and 523 clients were rehabilitated (Switzer, 1969).

Slowly, and sometimes contentiously, in bursts of major legislation the scope of public vocational rehabilitation was altered and its impact greatly enlarged. Client eligibility was expanded to include those who were mentally retarded or mentally ill, those with epilepsy, those socially handicapped as determined by a psychiatrist or psychologist, such as an adult public offender (Lassiter, 1972), and those who needed services to maintain their jobs. An emphasis on serving those with severe disabilities was mandated in the Rehabilitation Act of 1973 and in 1978, services were extended to those who did not have the potential for employment, but could benefit from services to live independently (Wright, 1980). Services themselves were broadened to include among others, physical restoration, maintenance expenses, and personal and social adjustment. Special grants were provided for the construction and operation of sheltered workshops, vocational evaluation and work adjustment centers, and other rehabilitation facilities (Lassiter, 1972). During fiscal year 1981 the federal government appropriated more than $800 million to the states on an 80/20, federal/state, matching basis. During that fiscal year more than 1 million clients were served and 255,881 were rehabilitated. These figures are down from the historical high of 361,138 clients rehabilitated during fiscal year 1974. The decline continued during the 1982 and 1983 fiscal years (RSA, 1982a, 1983, 1984).[7] Approximately 10,000 rehabilitation counselors served those clients in state agencies, a tremendous growth in personnel from the 143 rehabilitation workers in 1930 (Feinberg and McFarland, 1979; Wright, 1980).

The organization of the federal/state program of vocational rehabilitation has changed throughout its existence. In 1920 the federal agency assigned to administer the program was the Federal Board for Vocational Education, located in an education office. Various changes in the location and organization of the federal agency assigned to administer the program have occurred since then. By congressional mandate, in 1975 the administering agency, the Rehabilitation Services Administration (RSA), was placed within the Office of Human Development as a unit of what was then the Department of Health, Education and Welfare (Bitter, 1979). With the creation of the Department of Education in 1979, the Commissioner of RSA was legislated to report to the Assistant Secretary of the newly created Office of Special Education and Rehabilitation Services within the Department of Education (Wright, 1980).

The state agencies that administer the vocational rehabilitation programs have changed, too. Initially the programs were administered within state boards of education along with vocational education (Switzer, 1969). Federal legislation in 1954 permitted vocational rehabilitation agencies to move from those boards to other administrative agencies or to set up their own independent agency (Lassiter, 1972). The agency in which I did my research became a separate state agency with permanent status a few years after the 1954 federal legislation.

There are currently 56 state rehabilitation agencies, including those in the District of Columbia, Puerto Rico, Virgin Islands, American

Samoa, and Trust Territory. A total of 28 states have separate agencies for those who are blind (Bitter, 1979: 6), one of which is the state in which I did my research. My research does not focus on the state agency that serves those with severe visual impairments.

Rationale for Rehabilitation

The rationale for vocational rehabilitation is a combination of humanitarian concerns and economic benefits (Sussman, 1972). The relative emphasis on humanitarian concerns and economic benefits has changed over time, differs according to observers, and varies across rehabilitation professionals and, I suspect, agencies (Lassiter, 1972: 6).

Humanitarian concerns have provided an important rationale for vocational rehabilitation. Whether expressed in terms of "human dignity," the "value of every human being," the "right for self-expression and fulfillment," or "equality of opportunity," vocational rehabilitation has been based on an underlying concern for the person as an individual (McGowan, 1969; Sussman, 1972; Bitter, 1979).

The economic benefits of vocational rehabilitation have been readily recognized. From the "saving of trained manpower that otherwise would be lost" (Switzer, 1969: 40) to making people less dependent on the welfare state (Lassiter, 1972), to the economic returns to society in enabling individuals to become or remain employed (Sussman, 1972), the benefits to society of vocational rehabilitation have been stressed.[8] These benefits have been used often by proponents of vocational rehabilitation to back up humanitarian concerns when appealing for public support (Di Michael, 1969). Some observers feel the economic benefits have been the most salient justification for vocational rehabilitation (Switzer, cited in Lassiter, 1972; Sussman, 1972).

The emphasis on economic benefits may contradict humanitarian concerns and lead to practices that undermine those concerns (Sussman, 1972). The emphasis on economic returns may lead to fewer services provided more quickly to those most easily placed (Krause, 1965; Sinick, 1969; Lassiter, 1972). A "production-line practice of rehabilitation" may have grown out of the "long history of small, underpaid staffs, trying, with limited financial resources, to help large numbers of people cope with complicated rehabilitation problems" (Muthard, 1969: 276). Closed cases of successful rehabilitation may be a strongly emphasized goal to the extent that economic returns are stressed. And such a stress may strain rehabilitation counselors who believe they should be helping people but often find organizational policies sometimes seem to emphasize production at the possible expense of people. Within rehabilitation agencies, this issue is often expressed as the possible conflict between "quality" (of services) and "quantity" (the number served and successfully closed).

However, humanitarian and economic concerns need not be directly opposed to one another. On a general level, at which it is assumed that work is essential to human dignity, an emphasis on both concerns can be compatible (Di Michael, 1969; Lofquist, 1969). Thus the public program of vocational rehabilitation

> signifies the nation's recognition of its responsibility to provide disabled citizens with opportunities to be full participants in the world of work and the community in general [RSA, 1981:1].

Within the potential contradiction between humanitarian concerns and economic benefits and within other inconsistencies in society's response to those with disabilities (Bowe, 1978: 166-171) exist rehabilitation agencies and the work of rehabilitation counselors.[9]

CONCLUSION

Much of the work of vocational rehabilitation counselors, and more generally human service professionals, can be viewed usefully within the framework of detective work. Law enforcement detectives, rehabilitation counselors, and human service professionals gather, organize, and use information in order to meet their organizations' goals—solving crimes, rehabilitating individuals with impairments, or serving the needs of humans. To do that, each detective works cases, though what constitutes a case and how it is worked varies from organization to organization. Yet it is within those organizations that detective work is meaningful. Therefore, I turn my attention to the organization within which rehabilitation detectives work.

NOTES

1. The discussion about detective work, here and elsewhere, draws heavily on William B. Sanders's (1977) *Detective Work* and to a lesser, but still significant, extent on Skolnick (1966), Skolnick and Woodworth (1967), Sanders (1976, 1980), and Waegel (1981).

2. The roles of rehabilitation counselors—Are they counselors, coordinators, or perhaps clinicians?—and their functions have been debated, analyzed, and evaluated extensively (Whitehouse, 1975; Emener, 1978: 17-22; Rubin and Emener, 1979; Wright, 1980: 45-66).

3. We typically do not view detectives as providing services to individuals in the course of solving crimes, though solving crimes is, of course, a service to the community. However, detectives may informally provide services to victims (and even offenders) through advice, a friendly shoulder to lean on, or a sympathetic ear (Sanders, 1980: 91-94)

4. Counselors seem to be spending less time today in counseling and guidance (20% of their time in one study) than they did ten or fifteen years ago, when they spent approximately one-third of their time counseling and guiding. The time they do devote to counseling and guidance is less than they would like to devote (Rubin and Emener, 1979).

5. See the following for discussions of styles of vocational rehabilitation counseling and the effect of counseling on client outcomes: Bozarth et al. (1974), Bozarth and Rubin (1975), Bolton (1978), Emener (1978, 1980), Growick and Stueland (1979), Vandergroot and Engelkes (1980), Wright (1980), Ju (1982). A detailed analysis of "doing counseling and guidance" would likely require audio- or videotapes of what took place. See Erickson and Shultz (1982) for such an investigation of college counseling. To investigate counseling and guidance, one must first be clear as to what is and is not "C and G." A starting point would be to develop an understanding of what rehabilitation counselors understand C and G to be and when they are and are not doing it. Previous research has largely overlooked this issue.

6. For a more full discussion of the history of vocational rehabilitation, both public and private, see Obermann (1965), selections in Malikin and Rusalem (1969) and in Cull and Hardy (1972), Bitter (1979), and Wright (1980). Rehabilitation counseling in state vocational rehabilitation agencies is, of course, only part of rehabilitation counseling (Feinberg and McFarland, 1979).

7. The decline in clients rehabilitated seems attributable to the decline in purchasing power of rehabilitation dollars, which led to fewer clients served, and to a recent emphasis on serving the severely disabled individual (RSA, 1981). However, even the historically high number of clients served represents only a fraction, perhaps less than 10 percent, of those who could be eligible for services if services were more widely available, and funding conflicts continue (Bowe, 1980: chap. 4).

8. Benefit-cost ratios vary from study to study based on the assumptions made, calculations of the ratio, and the locale. Benefit-cost ratios higher than 40 to 1 have been calculated (Bitter, 1979: 5-6). The federal government estimates that for fiscal year 1980 the benefit-cost ratio is approximately 10 to 1: Estimated improved lifetime earnings are ten times the total costs on all closures (successful or not) during that year. In the last ten years that ratio has ranged from nearly 14 to 1 to 10 to 1 (RSA, 1981: 5-7: see also RSA, 1982b). However, government audits of state vocational rehabilitation agencies suggest that credit for rehabilitations is sometimes taken when it is not necessarily deserved (GAO, 1982). See Berkowitz et al. (1975) for a discussion of the difficulties in evaluating the economic benefits of rehabilitation.

9. The basic paradigm of rehabilitation is increasingly being questioned, particularly by those within the independent living movement. Those within the movement do not believe that the difficulties faced by those with disabilities are due primarily to their limitations. Instead, the difficulties are due to a social environment (of which rehabilitation is a part) that often limits and even oppresses individuals with disabilities. Consequently, those within the movement disagree with the rehabilitation paradigm about what should be done and how it should be done (DeJong, 1983).

2

THE REHABILITATION ORGANIZATION

Detectives, whether they be law enforcement, rehabilitation, or human service, work within organizations. Composed of policies, procedures, people, and the interplay among them, these organizations provide more than the settings for detectives in doing their work. Instead, the work of these detectives exists and becomes meaningful only within those organizations. For example, in order to solve crimes, detectives may get suspects to "cop out" to other offenses in addition to the one with which they are charged. In return, the suspects are not charged with the additional offenses, which would be likely to lead to reduced penalties. This practice of detectives' swapping reduced charges for suspects' confessions and thereby solving previously unsolved crimes becomes meaningful within law enforcement agencies that stress clearance rates (that is, the percentage of offenses known to police that they have "solved"; Skolnick, 1966: 167-181). Likewise, members of a psychiatric emergency team who make field visits in response to calls from the community might at times select the easiest cases for field visits instead of those that are most urgent. They might do so in order to dispose of cases quickly and return to paperwork or some other organizational responsibility (Emerson and Pollner, 1978). Detective work cannot be isolated from the organization in which it occurs. And, of course, the detectives not only work within those organizations, but they constitute an important feature of those organizations. To a great extent, particularly to the citizens with whom they come in contact, detectives *are* the organization (Lipsky, 1980: 13).

The rehabilitation counselors whom I observed worked in a nationally recognized *rehabilitation agency*. Like those nationwide, the agency confronted *policy* concerns of work, goals, and service, concerns that were paralleled by, though not identical to, the concerns of the *counselors.* And in responding to counselors' concerns within their agency's procedures and policies, counselors needed to address their (potential) *clients'* interests. Within this organizational interplay, rehabilitation work developed and became meaningful.

THE AGENCY

The state Vocational Rehabilitation Department, which allowed me to conduct my investigation, was nationally recognized as a leader in vocational rehabilitation.[1] Its network of fifteen area offices, each serving a different region of the state, and assorted rehabilitation facilities were considered a model for other agencies. As in other state agencies, a large variety of services were provided to its clients: evaluation, counseling and guidance, adjustment services, training, artificial appliances, job placement, and follow-up. And, as in other agencies, the one I observed served individuals with various impairments: mental illness and mental retardation, orthopedic impairments, digestive system disorders, hearing impairments, heart and circulatory conditions, genito-urinary system problems, cancer, and other impairments. The agency's staff constituted one of the largest chapters of a professional rehabilitation association.

The state Vocational Rehabilitation Department was one of the most successful rehabilitation agencies in the country. It ranked near the top in the number of clients served and rehabilitated per counselor and the number of severely disabled individuals rehabilitated per disabled population. The agency's operations were cost efficient and effective. Approximatley 95 percent of the rehabilitation dollars were spent for services to individuals. Those rehabilitation dollars paid big dividends in the form of increased earnings of the rehabilitated clients. Before rehabilitation, most of the clients were unemployed, a majority were dependent on family or friends for a living, and a significant percentage were in tax-supported institutions. After rehabilitation in a recent fiscal year, the rehabilitated clients were earning more than seven times as much at an annual rate as they had before rehabilitation.[2]

I observed one of the top area offices in the agency. It was a leader among the area offices in serving and rehabilitating individuals with vocationally handicapping impairments. Located in a major metropolitan area of the state, the office's rehabilitation counselors had a wide range of vocational rehabilitation programs and community resources to use in serving their clients. In doing their work, approximately thirty rehabilitation counselors drew upon the expertise of an area office supervisor, two quality control specialists, their own casework assistants, medical and psychological consultants, professional staff in the attached rehabilitation center, and community resources.[3]

Personnel

The area supervisor oversaw the area office. Serving as administrator, planner, trainer, evaluator, troubleshooter, and consultant, the supervisor had direct responsibility for the area office. As he noted in discussing one of his responsibilities, the training of staff:

> You can't expect people to do the job if you don't teach them how you want them to do the job. I think that is very important. I don't think we can depend on anybody else to do the training. I think that lies with me as to how I want this area run.

According to the philosophy and guidelines set by state administrators, the supervisor saw his responsibility as "interpreting those guidelines and trying to get the most out of those guidelines." Getting the most out of those guidelines meant that

> we ought to serve as many people as we can within the guidelines that we are working with, and be aggressive about it, and screening people in rather (than) screening people out for services . . . taking a more aggressive approach and maybe taking a few risks along the way, again within the guidelines and . . . in keeping my supervisor informed about what we are doing so I can have some guidepost to go by.

Through the implementation of state policy, assigning caseloads and territories for his counselors, managing financial resources, adjusting staffing patterns, handling complaints and questions, and in many other ways, the area supervisor influenced the activities of his counselors.[4]

Due to the large size of the area office, it had two quality control specialists. These two positions were staffed with rehabilitation professionals who each had approximately twenty years of experience with the agency and who had served previously as field counselors themselves. Just as the area supervisor had a wide range of responsibilities, so did the QCs, as the quality control specialists were called.[5] They (and the area office supervisor) led the case development staffings, group meetings among a handful of counselors to discuss the development of cases (see Chapter 5). They led a case manual study group for new counselors, reviewed almost all expenditures before the counselors authorized them, and provided day-to-day supervision of counselors' work. If difficulties or uncertainties arose regarding how to proceed, counselors came to them. All closures of cases and all plans developed on cases were reviewed by the QCs before they were sent to the state office to be reviewed.[6] Twice yearly the QCs audited the counselors' caseloads. As a state administrator remarked, the QC's responsibility was "to insure quality service to the clients."

Casework assistants aided rehabilitation counselors.[7] These assistants, all of whom were women in the local area office, had been called secretaries until relatively recently. The change in title was intended to reflect more clearly the importance of the assistants in the rehabilitation process. While the assistants ensured that the organization's appetite for the correct forms and paperwork was satisfied, they were much more than secretaries. They scheduled and rescheduled appointments of various kinds, administered some evaluation tests to the applicants, and were knowledgeable enough about the progress of cases to answer many questions should applicants or clients contact the office when the counselors were absent. Counselors often consulted assistants in deciding what to do next on a case, and some had formalized this procedure through regularly scheduled reviews of their cases with their assistants. New counselors repeatedly told me how invaluable the casework assistants were to them in orienting them to the job and their caseloads.

I did not examine the impact of casework assistants in rehabilitation detective work. To call them a "Dr. Watson" to the counselors' Sherlock Holmes does them an injustice, for they certainly did not serve as foils for their counselors' brilliant deductions. Instead, although their role was not completely clear to me, I know that they formed an important part of the detective work that led to those deductions.

A medical and a psychological consultant, the latter a full-time professional in the area office, the former a local doctor, provided both resources and obstacles for the counselors. By offering advice, recommendations, and diagnoses, the consultants provided resources for counselors to do their jobs. In many ways they served as the forensic, ballistic, and other technical experts whom detectives call upon in doing their work. However, the same advice, recommendations, and diagnoses at times were seen as obstacles by the counselors. The counselors were responsible, legally and practically, for the working of cases. However, the consultant's advice, recommendations, and diagnoses did not always support the counselors' views of their cases or what they had intended to do with them. Put simply, the consultants did not always say what the counselors wanted to hear. Thus how counselors consulted with the two consultants was important and will be pursued later.

A rehabilitation center, formerly called a workshop, provided vocational evaluation as well as personal, social, and work adjustment training for the counselors' applicants and clients. I did not investigate what takes place during adjustment training. No doubt those services were significant, but they were not provided by the counselors. However, how counselors may have used that training in working cases will be discussed later. Also, I did not systematically investigate the vocational evaluation provided by the rehabilitation center. When used, that evaluation was important in determining the vocational objective to be pursued by counselor and client. Depending on the caseload, client, and counselor, vocational evaluations at the rehabilitation center were more or less frequently used. Some counselors almost never referred their clients to the rehabilitation center, and other caseloads, such as those in the vocational rehabilitation public school programs, had their own evaluators. I decided to treat each of those evaluations as a "given"—information given to the counselors to be used in working cases—rather than a process to be investigated in its own right. How the counselors used such information is discussed later.[8]

Counselors also used the services of, as well as were constrained by, other professionals in rehabilitation and in the community. Doctors, psychologists, hearing aid dealers, proprietors of private training facilities (such as a barber school), school personnel, and others were important in affecting counselors' work. The staff of state rehabilitation facilities, such as those dealing with alcohol problems, were also important. Again, what actually takes place within those agencies or between clients and the community professionals does not concern me here. How counselors dealt with some of those agencies and professionals in doing their own jobs, however, does interest me.

Location and Layout

During the course of my research, the local area office moved to a new facility, but a small contingent of personnel—several counselors, assistants, and a quality control specialist—remained in the original area office. The new area office, along with the new, attached rehabilitation center, was located several miles from downtown and from the original office. It was located "across the river," a place where some clients had rarely ventured previously.

The local area office also had a suboffice located in a county seat of one of the several counties served by the area office. The intent was to serve more effectively and efficiently a fairly concentrated population within the geographical region served by the area office, but which was sufficiently distant from the area office to make service from the area office difficult. The concentration of the population justified a suboffice. I did not examine the rehabilitation work of the counselors in this suboffice.

Several vocational rehabilitation public school programs were administered by the area office. The public school programs were usually located at a public high school or other school facility. Project supervisors had reponsibility for managing the programs as well as carrying out their own counseling responsibilities. I will discuss the former responsibility but not the latter. Finally, one field counselor was responsible for handling cases that developed out of workers compensation claims. The location of these "satellite" offices had some impact on counselors' work. For example, the commuting distances between these and the main offices at times led to most of an afternoon being used for a relatively great deal of driving to get to short meetings.

While the physical layouts of the two area office facilities and the public school programs differed in many specific ways, the general features were similar. The major distinction, particularly in the two area offices, was between private (counselors' and other staff's) and public (clients') space. Each of the offices had a waiting area for the clients, which to a great degree screened them visually from the private offices of the counselors and the less private work stations of the assistants. Clients remained in the waiting area until called for by counselors or their assistants. A large conference room was the setting for areawide and other meetings of counselors and staff. A similar room had served that function in the original office. "Break rooms" with coffee pots or vending machines were available in the two main offices. Staff might eat their lunches in that room or take short breaks there in the morning and afternoon.

The physical layout of the offices had some important consequences for the counselors' work. For example, the distinction between private and public spaces, the existence of an "inner sanctum" (the counselor's office), and the procedure of clients' waiting to be ushered "back" to see the counselors enabled counselors to control more effectively the flow of their work.[9] The side-by-side arrangement of offices, the common hallways, and the break rooms facilitated, even encouraged, counselors to discuss their work, both specific cases as well as the larger world of rehabilitation work. Of course, conversation unrelated to work was encouraged by these arrangements as well. In its most obvious manifestations—offices, desks, chairs, file cabinets, telephones, and the like—the agency's facilities provided a secure, professional setting in which counselors did their work. The subtle importance of the physical features of the agency became apparent when counselors left their offices in the course of their work, a matter to be discussed in the following chapters (see Lipsky, 1980: 117-118).

Caseloads

In order to serve clients and administer the rehabilitation program effectively, the agency, like other human service organizations (Gell, 1969; McCleary, 1978), operated using caseloads. Each field counselor had responsibility for at least one caseload. A few had responsibility for two small ones. These caseloads were structured according to the kind of disability/client served and/or the geographical territory the caseload encompassed. Counselors who handled a general caseload served clients with a wide range of vocationally handicapping conditions. Others managed a specialty caseload, in which clients had a particular, defining characteristic. In the area office, specialty caseloads involved clients with hearing impairments, public offenders, the public school programs, clients who had filed Workers Compensation cases with the state's Industrial Commission, and four that were dissolved before I ended my research: one involving clients with epilepsy, one concerning clients involved in CETA (the Comprehensive Employment Training Act), Supplemental Security Income (SSI) recipients, and Social Security Disability Insurance (SSDI) recipients (Bitter, 1979: 224-225). In large measure they were dissolved due to changes in federal involvement with the programs. Some of these specialty caseloads, such as the hearing impaired caseload, had almost exclusive jurisdiction over clients with the distinguishing characteristic and, in turn, were limited to such clients. Other specialty caseloads did not have such exclusive jurisdiction.

Some counselors who officially worked a general caseload specialized in certain kinds of cases either "exclusively" or to a great extent. These involved primarily clients with drug problems, particularly alcohol abuse, clients with mental health problems, or public offenders. This nondesignated specialization was officially recognized. Other counselors, particularly those with a general caseload, might handle clients with the above disabilities or characteristics, but did not specialize in such cases. Thus caseloads varied as to whether or not they were restricted to clients with certain kinds of disabilities or special characteristics. After the four specialty caseloads had been dissolved, approximately two-fifths of the caseloads in the area office were designated as specialty caseloads and two-thirds of those were public school caseloads.

The possible parallel between specialty caseloads within rehabilitation counseling and specialty details within detective work, such as juvenile, burglary, and major crimes, may have already become apparent. In Chapter 6, I explore the parallel as well as the specific workings of several specialty caseloads.

Caseloads were also based on territories. These were geographical subregions within the larger geographical area served by the area office. Counselors who managed a general caseload were assigned territories, which served as a geographical source of clients. While exceptions were made for the convenience of the clients, clients were served typically by counselors assigned to the territory in which the clients lived. Those who worked public school caseloads were also assigned territories or developed them on their own. In these situations territories consisted of public high schools.[10]

POLICY

The vocational rehabilitation program in America is goal oriented. Whether this is a strength (Bitter, 1979: 37) or a weakness (Krause, 1965) depends in large part on what is meant by "goal oriented" and how that concept is implemented. Nationwide, the rehabilitation program aims to achieve a desired end: the successful employment of individuals with vocationally handicapping impairments. Services are not merely given away, but are provided to reach a specific goal.

However, when justifying a program's existence to the public and particularly to funding sources, an emphasis on a seemingly objective and easily quantified aspect of the goal may develop. Rehabilitation programs, like other human service agencies, must show evidence to regulatory/funding agencies of what they are doing. Hard data—numbers concerning clearance rates (Skolnick, 1966: 167-181), placement rates (Blau, 1955: 36-56), case services (Altheide and Johnson, 1980: chaps. 4, 5), and other data nowadays seem to be preferred in documenting what is being done by an agency:

> Regulatory and/or funding agents and agencies see numbers as the most efficient means of weighing what is spent in service institutions and for communicating what is accomplished for clients. Institutional administrators and accounting officers support the claim of efficiency, which underpins their growing interest in the hard data products of behavioral treatment strategies [Gubrium and Buckholdt, 1979: 116].

However, the relationship between "hard" data and "soft" services may be problematic at best (Lipsky, 1980: 167).

Successful closures, known as "26s," traditionally have represented the hard data in vocational rehabilitation. Rehabilitation professionals have become increasingly concerned about the inadequacy and the dysfunctions of merely counting the number of cases in which the clients become successfuly employed in order to assess counselors' and agencies' performances. Such hard data are inadequate because they overlook the varying complexities of clients' situations, services rendered, and clients' outcomes (Reagles et al., 1971; Rubin and Cooper, 1977; Crisler and Edwards, 1980; Wright, 1980). They are dysfunctional because they may lead to "creaming" (skimming the most easily served clients from those more difficult to serve), quick rather than thorough evaluation and provision of services, finessing of eligibility, inappropriate but quick placement, falsification of records, and other activities that make counselors and agencies "look good," but do not necessarily serve those with the greatest need (Walls and Moriarity, 1977; GAO, 1978, 1982; Couch, 1979; Smits and Ledbetter, 1979; Vernon et al., 1979). Quality becomes sacrificed perhaps for quantity. While alternatives have been suggested, "26" closures remain the hard data for assessing counselors' and agencies' performances.

Thus a "goal orientation" has partially become an emphasis on "meeting your goals." An orientation has become objectified into something that is quantified. And with counting come some practices that seem to be at odds with the original orientation of the agencies (Lipsky, 1980: 48-53), whether those agencies are vocational rehabilitation departments, employment agencies (Blau, 1955: 36-56), psychiatric emergency teams (Emerson and Pollner, 1978), or detective details within law enforcement departments (Skolnick, 1966: 167-181).

Work

Similar concerns that existed nationwide also existed in the state vocational rehabilitation department and the local area office I observed. The agency's goal was to enable individuals with impairments to work successfully; that was its mandate. Consequently, administrators were concerned when federal legislation was proposed that would lump funding of their program with social service and welfare programs into block grants to the states. A letter-writing campaign to federal legislators was undertaken to oppose the proposal. Such legislation, which was not approved, to the relief of the agency and of others nationwide, was partly seen as seriously jeopardizing the mission of rehabilitation, which was to help people with disabilities to work.

The agency stressed this mission. However painful the decisions were, they were not "in the business of saving lives" (though their services did so at times). A quality control specialist made that difficult point when discussing a counselor's desire to work with a client who suffered from near-end-stage renal disease.

> But, you know, we really have to think in terms: what are we doing? Is it vocational rehabilitation, or is it a good thing to do in extending life? That's what the doctors do. We have to look at it, remember, in vocational rehabilitation. In other words, get the person back to employment. We have to look at it in such a way that hopefully that this person is, repaid [The counselor: (his) debt to society]. That's right, that's right . . . but keep all those things in mind during this period. Not only just determining what he can do. But let's look at: Is he going to be able to do it? Is he going to be here to do it? [The QC and the case development staffing group decided to do an extended evaluation (up to 18 months) in order to determine a vocational objective and follow the clients' progress.]

To a question regarding the agency's serving cancer patients whose prognosis was eight to ten months, which was raised by physical therapists at a local hospital where a counselor was explaining the vocational rehabilitation program, the counselor responded:

> Well, we might be able to get involved, [but] if you [the therapists] are simply working with them [the terminally ill patients] and then discharging them [to] "go home to die," we really wouldn't be involved.

Goals

As in all such agencies, "goal oriented" also meant meeting your goals. The rehabilitation professionals were expected to produce. Counselors were assigned goals—a specific number of successful closures and rehabilitation plans—to be attained each fiscal year (from July 1 to June 30 of the following year). Just as nationwide the number of successful rehabilitations and clients served has been decreasing, the goals set for the counselors by the state administrators had been decreasing, too. In the recent past, goals for successful closures were as high as 95; now they have decreased to approximately 60 for a general caseload.[11]

Monthly reports distributed to the counselors and supervisory staff showed how well counselors and their colleagues were doing in the local area office and statewide. Comparisons among them could be made easily. Similar production reports are used in other human service agencies. In one public welfare department, the report was called "the fink sheet" because it informed on the social workers who were not performing well (Altheide and Johnson, 1980: 140).

Counselors' progress toward these goals was monitored by the area supervisory staff and state administrators. Monitoring was as casual as the area supervisor's walking past a counselor and asking how well the plans and closures were going. It became more formal as the end of the fiscal year approached. As one counselor noted in mid-June, the upcoming staff meeting on Monday of the following week would be the last time the area supervisor could "get on us" to get those closures. This was not said in condemnation. Counselors were consulted regarding how they expected to do by the end of the fiscal year, were encouraged to do their best, and were asked for tentative closure and plan totals. At one area-wide meeting, counselors were informed the area office would come up short in meeting their goals, but that if counselors turned in the number of closures they had "promised," then the shortfall would not be too great. During the course of my research, this more formal monitoring was increased to every three months. The intent was to follow more closely counselors' progress toward their goals so action could be taken, if necessary, before it was too late. A counselor "testified" to this quarterly monitoring, for he had fallen behind in closures a few months into a new fiscal year. For several weeks he primarily "worked on closures" so he could "catch up."

Production levels were used to justify positions and programs. After a relatively successful year, the area office supervisor noted at a staff meeting that, while there might be layoffs in the agency because of the state government's "belt tightening," due to their high level of production relative to other area offices, their area office would be at the bottom of the list for any future reduction in staff. However, warning notices would be sent in the future to counselors who were not producing. Those who were not producing ran the risk of being terminated. At an earlier meeting, the supervisor noted that low-producing caseloads might be dissolved and the counselors assigned to those caseloads could be reassigned to other caseloads, perhaps in other cities. A quality control specialist remarked to the counselors he supervised that if the counselors kept up the level of referrals, plans, and successful closures, they could then justify the present number of assistants they had. Yearly performance appraisals were based partly on production, too.

Production levels were used to justify entire programs as well. In explaining the difficulties of justifying a new vocational rehabilitation school program in which school-age clients were likely to be served several years before being successfully closed, a project supervisor noted:

> This is the problem we have had convincing the state office that we are working over here. The first year, I had no closures. Because when you pick up cases, we picked up forty or some odd cases that year, but we had very few to graduate. There were none that were going to graduate. If they did, these were of the higher caliber students, and some of them were going to college. So that was an additional four years. But yet I still had a number that I had to meet. There was no way we could meet goals over here. . . . [The area supervisor] said, "Hey, give him just a little time." It has taken a couple of years for the turnover and [as the cases do turn over] we double our closure every year over here.

Production was also important in reassigning personnel from one position or caseload to another. An adjustment specialist who had recently become a field counselor explained:

As a VR adjustment specialist I was doing so much placement, which is not typically the responsibility [of the adjustment specialist]. I don't really know of any other work adjustment or personal, social, work adjustment program where an adjustment specialist was so interested. And my last two months there, I think I placed eighteen folks in jobs. And I wasn't really being accountable for that because I had all the other responsibilities. And I think our area supervisor realized those were my strengths, and he called me in one day and said, "How would you like to be a counselor?"

Particular counselors were assigned to certain caseloads because those caseloads produced well. If those caseloads had been left temporarily vacant, or if less effective counselors had been assigned to them, then their productivity would have suffered.

This concern with production became expressed symbolically near the end of my intensive observations, when the agency and the area office adopted a "marketing" approach in their work. The agency was to market both itself and its clients to the employment community. Counselors became responsible for developing formal contacts with employers to discover the employers' needs and how the agency might meet those needs. For example, perhaps "troubled" employees could be helped. Counselors were to develop job leads and share them with fellow counselors who constituted their marketing team. Counselors became the liaisons between the employers and the agency. On-site training opportunities for some of the agency's clients were developed. Once clients were rehabilitated, they were to be "marketed" as qualified workers, not as individuals with impairments. While some of the staff questioned whether the approach was "all that new," the term itself symbolically emphasized the importance of production.

The symbolism of production has appeared in other human service agencies. One official in a state department of corrections remarked,

> The DC is a business. The problems and solutions are the same. Our customer is the public and our product is parolees. Most POs [parole officers] don't care enough about the customer and certainly not enough about product quality [McCleary, 1978: 47]

Being one of the most successful state vocational rehabilitation departments in the country, the agency's and area office's pride in their results was evident. Annual reports for public dissemination depicted pictorially the number of clients served and the number rehabilitated in counties throughout the state. The statewide total was proclaimed in bold-type numerals. After a successful year in comparison to other area offices, one counselor in the area office I observed noted to a quality control specialist that their supervisor must have been grinning at the recent meeting of area office supervisors; pride followed production.

Service

Just as there was nationwide concern about the potential dysfunctions of "counting closures," there was also concern in the state agency I observed. With the appointment of new state administrators in the mid-1970s, the agency took stock of its practices. And as one of those administrators remarked, "Frankly, we were not overly thrilled." The administrators were concerned about the quality of services provided and the impact those services had on the clients. Too often, the agency was merely paying a bill—surgical, dental, medical or eyeglass—without rendering other significant services directly. With rising medical costs and the requirement of the Rehabilitation Act of 1973 to give priority to serving those who are severely disabled, the administrators "deliberately" and "methodically" began to cut back on cases that solely involved physical restoration or medical follow-up. Through discussion, persuasion, and "hellacious arguments" among the state office staff; through the complete revision of the case service manual for counselors and the manual for the casework assistants; through conferences, workshops, and in-service training for professional staff; and through careful audits of counselors' caseloads and discussion of the findings with area supervisors and the counselors, the administrators attempted to implement the change in policy consistently and thoroughly.

For an agency that was more than fifty years old, such a change was not made overnight, and not without some discomfort. As the administrator noted, the changes

> traumatized a lot of our staff. In fact, we had a lot of counselors who just couldn't understand what we were doing—why—and quit, retired early . . . . It has been an awful few years for some of us. . . we've fired a few folks and we've urged some retirements of a few folks.

But in being persistent, the administrators

knocked physical restoration in the head, and said to folks, if all they need is that—a bill paid—then they've come to the wrong place.

No longer could the "three Hs"—hernia, hysterectomy, and hemorrhoids—which typically involved only surgery, be the primary basis for eligibility (Vernon et al., 1979: 45-46). No longer would the following incident, which occurred in another state, be acceptable (if it ever would have been acceptable) in the agency I observed:

> A welfare recipient was admitted to one of the hospitals and had her gallstones removed. Her hospitalization was paid by Medicaid, and the State rehabilitation agency paid for the surgery. The patient received no other services from the State rehabilitation agency, and was still on welfare when the counselor closed her case as "successfully rehabilitated" [GAO, 1978: 58].

No longer would counselors merely purchase eyeglasses, dental work, or medical follow-up (visits to a physician and medication) as the only service provided to clients.

Instead, with the change in agency policy came the emphasis on the agency's professional, *substantial involvement* in the rehabilitation of its clients. According to the agency's revised manual:

> throughout the provision of services, he (the counselor) must maintain close contact with the client to see that the rehabilitation process is not interrupted. Services must progress in an orderly manner and on a timely basis in order to be successful.

Further, the services

> provided by this agency and its agents must be above and beyond those already available to all persons and not otherwise attainable from other sources.

As a quality control specialist noted in explaining to me what he needed to check when a case was submitted to him for successful closure:

> What I have to look at . . . is: Have we provided meaningful services? Have we really had some impact into this case? Is it such that if we had not intervened, and [I'm] not thinking in terms of paying the bill for the medical thing, but if we had not intervened, is there a possibility that this person may not be employed now or may not be employed successfully?

Or, as stated more concretely by the other quality control specialist in a case development staffing:

> Anytime we have a disability, and we can show guidance and counseling and job placement, that's substantial services. It better be . . . or we are going to be in trouble.

However, the meaning of substantial involvement/services in practice, not just in policy, must await the analysis of rehabilitation detective work in the following chapters.

With the change in the rehabilitation agency's policy, the *service* in that human service agency was stressed once again. However, counting closures retained its importance in the agency, though the number of closures to be counted decreased. The relative emphasis on quantity and quality shifted. Yet counselors were still expected to serve both masters. To do so was not always easy; how this was done is discussed in the following chapters.

REHABILITATION COUNSELORS

Like other human service professionals, rehabilitation counselors work within organizations. While the counselors' concerns may not be identical to the administration's concerns, the counselors cannot ignore them (see Lipsky, 1980: 16-25). Within those organizational concerns, counselors do their work while developing a perspective of it. The latter concerns me here. Organizational concerns were paralleled by, though not identical to, the concerns of the counselors: work, goals, and service.

Work

Many times I heard counselors say vocational rehabilitation was not a "giveaway" program. As one counselor remarked in discussing future clients who might want a service, such as dental work, on which the agency was cutting back: "They're going to find out that we're not a giveaway program. . . . We're a work program." Another counselor told an inquiring individual in a telephone conversation that rehabilitation was not "welfare," that the aim of the rehabilitation agency was to enable people to become gainfully employed. Once employed, their tax dollars could be used to support the program. Similar remarks were used by counselors in their initial contact with prospective clients. The use of such remarks will be explored later. A third counselor resented the possibility of being lumped with social services in the public's mind and in federal funding.

The agency's mandate and emphasis on getting clients back to work was the reason one counselor felt the agency was a good one, perhaps the best in the state:

> I think we are the best because . . . if the job is done right, we do more to get more people back out into the mainstream . . . of the world of what's going on. I don't care what type problem you got—if it's alcohol, mental illness—if you ain't working, then you[r] problem's bigger. The one thing I always try to emphasize at the [facility] . . . you can be crazy, but if you are putting in a salary, if you are not too crazy, the family is going to tolerate. But the day you lose that money and there ain't none coming in and you are sitting around and you become a burden on the other people, then your behavior becomes deviant. I've seen it happen so many times. I think we, more than anybody else if we do our job right, can do more to help people get back into that [work] than . . . all the medications and mental hospitals and all the alcohol treatment. Along with those things, if we can help put that final thing there, then we've really done something. We can do that type thing more than anybody else. Plus using the resources of them all. I'm not downing on none of the agencies [laughter]. But I just think we are probably closer to helping somebody do this.[12]

Counselors' personal beliefs in the "work ethic" (Thomas et al., 1974), the agency's emphasis on getting clients back to work, and its concern with counselors' producing combined to help shape counselors' views toward clients and their attempts or lack of attempts to work. Many counselors could not understand and were upset that some of their clients showed so little interest in working. These counselors' concerns about their clients' and potential clients' lack of desire to work have been echoed nationwide (Bitter and Kunce, 1972; Salomone, 1972; Zadny and James, 1976, 1979b). Its significance in rehabilitation detective work is discussed later.

Conversely, counselors admired those individuals who wanted to work no matter how difficult the situation might be. When asked to comment in a staffing about a counselor's applicant whose wife had left him, who had been fired from several jobs in a row, and who had "crying spells" but wanted job placement assistance from the agency, another counselor remarked:

> Well, I would be most interested to know how he is coping with these things other than crying. You know, the family broken down, no job. And he still wants to work. That's interesting, too. I mean he has lost all his jobs and he still wants to work. I kinda admire that fellow.

As I discuss later, that admiration also influenced counselors' work.

Goals

Among law enforcement detectives, "stats" are often, but not universally, important (Skolnick, 1966: 167-181; Sanders, 1977; Waegel, 1981). Arrests and clearances may be seen by detectives as important elements to be used in assessing their performance. In one department

> most detectives believe that the crude number of lockups they make is used as a basis for assessing their performance and competence in doing investigative work. Every arrest a detective makes is entered into a logbook, which is available for inspection by superiors and from which they can compare each detective's arrest level with that of others.
>
> Ambitious detectives in particular are very conscious of producing a steady stream of arrests, feeling that this is an effective way to achieve recognition and promotion [Waegel, 1981: 267].

In many ways the above could be said of rehabilitation counselors and other human service professionals (for example, see Blau, 1955).

While counselors took pride in their agency's work orientation, they fully realized the importance of "meeting their goals." One counselor mentioned that "numbers were important," but that if I repeated what she said, she would deny having said it. What was the big secret? There was none. As one counselor explained about meeting goals:

> Oh, it's something we think about every day.... It's something that from July 1 to June 30 is something that's constantly in the forefront. It's something that if you want to be a successful counselor, you are going to live with.

Another counselor noted that she thought about goals constantly, even during the initial contact with a prospective client: Would this prospective client become a "26" or not?

Out of the counselors' (well-founded) concern with goals came an emphasis on monitoring their own progress toward their goals. Many divided their yearly goals into monthly ones so they could gauge their gradual progress or lack thereof. As one counselor noted:

> I really take that sort of thing seriously. I try to break it down month by month. My goal is seventy, so if we can get like six or seven closures a month, that we would pretty much have it made. But months I only get two or three, it really bothers me.

Counselors compared how well they were doing in the present fiscal year with how they had done at comparable points in the past fiscal year. Being ahead or behind last year's pace was an indication of one's progress, too. Counselors would check monthly reports to see if the official totals matched their own. One counselor checked each month with his QC to make sure none of his plans or closures had been "lost"—had gone unrecorded. When assessing their progress, counselors would count on particular clients becoming 26s and were disappointed if something happened that resulted in "failure." Concern with goals grew as the end of the fiscal year approached. That concern affected the counselors' activities, a subject discussed in Chapter 5.

The end of the fiscal year brought to the office a mixture of satisfaction, disappointment with renewed determination, and lament. Many took satisfaction in meeting or exceeding their goals. Some looked forward to the new fiscal year as a chance to start fresh. With renewed determination (and, they hoped, with clients whose cases would soon be closed in July or August, thus providing a good start) they would meet their goals. However, others lamented the fact that on July 1 their previous "successess" had been "wiped off" the tally; they would be starting from zero again.

While the organizational significance of goals was widely recognized by counselors, and, in turn, counselors generally endowed goals with personal significance for their work, their feelings toward that impor-tance varied. Collectively, the mix of feelings was widely shared, though the relative emphasis on particular feelings varied among the counselors. Not too surprisingly, counselors generally wished there was less emphasis on goals, in particular they wished the number was lowered. As one remarked, "Well, I don't think anybody likes the idea of feeling that kind of pressure." However, counselors realized that the importance of goals had not been "sprung on" them:

And before I accepted the job I was told this during the inteview that, you know, we are goal oriented. It was not like a slap in my face, [as if] I didn't know what I was getting into before accepting the position.

Goals were viewed as potential obstacles in providing greater services to clients (Krause, 1965). The importance of numbers typically led to large caseloads with more than 100 people being worked with at any one time, though more than 200 was not unusual in the recent past.[13] With such large caseloads, counselors felt that they just did not have the time to provide more and lengthier counseling sessions or greater on-the-job follow-up (Emener and Rubin, 1980).[14] Other human service professionals face similar constraints (Prottas, 1979: 21).

While goals were seen as potential obstacles to serving clients, counselors viewed them as a useful criterion for evaluating their performance:

I don't like the quota that you have got so many to do. However, it is just like it is a motivator. It's sort of a measurement. It is not a true measurement, but it is somewhat of a measurement of what you are doing.

*　　　　　*　　　　　*

I really think if people look at ratings of counselors and looked at their goals and looked at their work, they would be more closely related than people would like to say that they are. But everybody fusses about them. But I just think—I think you've got to have something to show, you know, the closures—you've got to have something to show the work you do. You know, sometimes it gets a little too carried away. You know, but you need, even if [it] wasn't as it is . . . you still got to have something to say, "Yeah, I've accomplished this."

While some counselors wondered whether they and their colleagues would do less work if there were no goals, in other states goals have been found to be strongly related to the number of clients successfully rehabilitated (Zadny and James, 1979a).

Due to self-selection into and out of the agency, socialization within the agency, and accommodation to the agency, counselors accepted goals with more or less equanimity. Goals were an important, if not completely desirable, feature of the agency confronted by counselors. However, few counselors were as seemingly nonchalant as the following counselor, though even her remarks indicate the adaptation counselors make to the specter of goals:

> I used to hate them, used to be angry having them. Now, I just really don't pay much attention to them anymore. I'm going to get them [the agency] what I can get.[15]

Because goals were important, counselors justified why they could not, would not, or had not met them. Although I was not the audience who mattered, counselors often expressed their justifications to me. These varied from being assigned to a caseload during the fiscal year, to leaves of absence (such as maternity or medical) to new caseloads taking time to become established and productive, to the inability of the caseload itself to produce such goals, to the current state of the economy. One counselor noted that she did not mind the goals for rehabilitation plans, but she did not feel she was in complete control of closures:

> I feel like I can do—I can generate the types of things that will get plans. But the closures, you know, I feel much less comfortable about the closures goal. [Why?] Because like people can quit their jobs, and you can't do anything to make them stop that. [In other words, it's a little bit out of your control.] It's out of your control. It really is. And also some of our clients, you know, you may have all the motivation in the world for that person to go back to work, but the person is not really motivated . . . there is a lot of people we can't make go to work.

While the counselor quoted above lamented her lack of control over clients' going to work, that is, of course, the agency's goal. In trying to achieve that goal, counselors do attempt to control what happens with their clients. How they do so is discussed in the following chapters.

With goals being a pervasive concern in the agency and among counselors, the counselors were aware of and concerned in varying degrees, with how their colleagues were doing during the present fiscal year and had done in past years. Consequently, some friendly rivalries, admiration, and even contempt developed among the counselors. Two counselors kept each other posted on the number of applicants they had received, plans they had developed, and clients whose cases had been closed successfully. Counselors pointed in admiration to some of their colleagues whose performances were outstanding, who "ripped the devil out of goals," or who had good attitudes and attained their goals. Others, however, might be seen as not pulling their weight. It was the "top producers" who were carrying them and the office. Thus counselors made comparisons among one another that were based in part upon their relative production.

Service

Rehabilitation counselors brought to the organization a concern for people. When asked how they became rehabilitation counselors, they typically answered that they were interested in working with people, wanted to help others, got hooked through acquaintances who were involved in human services, or the like. One counselor responded:

I guess when I was really in high school. I really didn't know what VR was all about. I had a friend who was a paraplegic. And we were very close, and just me, being me, I have always liked to interact with people and just loved people.

Counselors characterized themselves as "people oriented" or as "needing to work with people." One counselor had previously worked for the Disability Determination Division of the agency, which determines eligibility for disability payment from the Social Security Administration. The position involved primarily paperwork. The counselor remarked:

I had heard that rehab, you know, it is a growing agency.... So I decided to try and get in with them. And it was with Disability Determination. They needed some people. So I went over and got on with them at DDD. And thinking this was going to be the thing. You know, won't have to see people and do everything just from paper. I stayed there, went through [the] training period, and I stayed there about six months. I had not said anything, but secretly I was ready to go back to employment services. I was ready to go anywhere and get back among the living again. I can't handle, I can't just stick to papers. I didn't like it.

Counselors derived satisfaction from their work in helping people, making a difference in their clients' lives, even if they received relatively little recognition from the clients or the agency (Sussman and Haug,

1970). In discussing one client he considered to be a "success story," a counselor stated:

> That's what it's all about. It's taking a person like that and just being involved with them and helping them to do the things that they want to do and giving them the opportunities to do it.

Even if the success was short-lived, knowing one's involvement was making some difference could be exhilarating. As a counselor who had been on the job just a few months said:

> I don't know, it's exciting to think that, you know, you go through a case with a kid, or there's been a couple of clients that I've had a lot of real close contact with, and, uh, there is a lot of disappointments already, you know, with a couple of them. But I've really enjoyed just, just knowing that one of them got a job. I got a phone call today that he lost it the second day, but, but yet it was a really good feeling when he got it because you feel like you've been in there plugging.

And as another counselor noted, what he and other counselors do can "touch so many lives," not just those of the clients.

Being people oriented, counselors welcomed the agency's recent shift in policy away from paying bills and toward greater substantial involvement in the clients' rehabilitation. As one counselor noted,

> Rehab counselors for a while where arrangers, doing more arranging than they were doing counseling. I feel like now we are more into what we should be doing than what we were doing in the past.

Another counselor remarked,

> I think most counselors feel real positive about the change. The fact that they're able to use the training that they've had in order to really work with clients, to get out and really place clients.

Some counselors, however, questioned which activities were to be considered substantial services and which were not. One counselor questioned whether "vision cases" should be eliminated. The counselor explained:

> I feel very strongly that sometimes we are weeding out cases that we should work with. For example, [name of individual] is [position held in

the agency].... He wears glasses. If he met economic need and came over here and we opened a case on him [and] he didn't have his glasses. His vision is 20/200 without his glasses, but corrected to like 20/20, perfect vision. Okay, our manual states that unless we have a 25 percent loss or a 35 percent, anyway, we cannot provide glasses as a primary disability. And if [name] had no other disability that would be primary, then we could not assist him. And that is wrong. Without his glasses, he is blind . . . but with his glasses, it alleviates the handicap.

Another counselor wondered how much difference there was between the visual and dental cases in which the agency was becoming less involved and those that involved clients with hearing impairments in which the agency was maintaining its involvement. While some counselors broadly questioned what should or should not be considered substantial services, it was the establishment of need for substantial services and documentation that it had been provided in particular cases that concerned counselors on an everyday basis.

Although counselors were people oriented, they worked within an agency that also stressed meeting your goals. Thus, to varying degrees, they were ambivalent about the new policy. Many claimed it had no impact on their work; they served clients who were being provided substantial services. They had not been to any significant extent "bill-paying" counselors. These same counselors suggested that other counselors, particularly those who managed a general caseload, might be experiencing difficulties. As one counselor responded to my inquiry about the possible impact of the new policy on counselors' meeting their goals:

And that has affected goals for the year, and I think probably added more pressure to counselors who are trying to get their goals for the year, because naturally we did have cases that were quick-turnover cases, whether they be dental, hernia, anybody that was at that point, if you could provide, say, an operation that client really needed in order to continue working, and maybe he was already working. Well, see, you didn't have to get involved in job placement. The client was already working. So that was an immediate quick-turnover case. So goals have been hurt to a certain degree, or at least it's put more pressure to get the goals, I think.

However, at the end of the fiscal year in which the change in policy had been primarily implemented, the area supervisor noted that the transition had gone well. Only two or three caseloads greatly concerned him. While the transition seemed to have gone smoothly in the area office I observed, counselors knew of other area offices where the transition was proving more difficult. And, as noted earlier, according to a state administrator, the change traumatized some counselors. It was, however, a change to which all who remained had to adapt.

THE CLIENTS

What is missing in this description of the rehabilitation organization are the clients. Yet clients have a profound effect on the behavior of human service professionals, and in turn, their behavior "has a profound effect on the implementation of public policy" (Prottas, 1979: 163). Whether clients are demanding or acquiescent, knowledgeable or ignorant, resourceful or resourceless, or possess other characteristics and engage in other behaviors can intentionally and unintentionally affect the behavior of human service professionals. The professionals' responses to clients' behavior becomes the everyday implementation of their agencies' public policies. For example, youthful suspects who are civil toward police officers are less likely to be arrested than are antagonistic suspects (Lundman et al., 1978). Moreover, welfare workers "freely admit that they sometimes process unpleasant clients out of turn to avoid seeing them repeatedly and to avoid explaining the delays invariably associated with the routine procedure" (Prottas, 1979: 109). Thus, through the responses of human service professionals to the "presentations" of their (potential) clients, agency and public policy becomes implemented.

Experienced rehabilitation counselors were well aware of the importance of clients for their own work. Without clients they would be out of work, but not just any kind of client would work out. Based on training and experience, counselors developed general perspectives about clients. For example, counselors routinely stated that people cannot be rehabilitated against their will, which was more descriptively stated as "you can't squeeze blood from a turnip." During the course of individual cases, counselors developed views about those with whom they were working. For example, a counselor might decide that a particular client had little intention of seriously seeking employment. Those general perspectives, as well as specific characterizations of clients developed by counselors during the course of cases influenced how counselors did their work. How those perspectives and characterizations did so is examined in the following chapters.

And, of course how (potential and actual) clients presented themselves to the agency made a difference, too. Some, though not all, clients were ignorant of the agency's procedures and services. Some presented well-articulated desires, while others had little desire at all. Typically, clients came to the agency voluntarily, though some were required to participate by other agencies and others believed services were not available elsewhere. Some sought to be served by the agency, others perhaps to "use" it. Counselors responded to these and other presentations. However, the agency's policy and procedures and their own concerns needed to be addressed as well.

CONCLUSION

Detectives, whether law enforcement, rehabilitation, or human service, work within organizations, and their work becomes understandable only within those organizations. The rehabilitation counselors whom I observed worked in a nationally regarded state agency that was both goal and service oriented. The agency served vocationally handicapped individuals in order to enable them to remain or become successfully employed. To demonstrate its success in doing so, the professional staff were expected to produce, and the agency stressed reaching its goal. However, with a new administration and nationwide concern that an emphasis on quantity had undermined quality, the agency revised its policy to stress substantial services to its clients. Out of societal concerns that may be contradictory or inconsistent— humanitarian concerns and economic benefits in the case of rehabilitation (see Chapter 1)—organizational goals develop that may conflict as well (Lipsky, 1980).

Within the rehabilitation agency's concerns of work, goals, and service, counselors developed similar, though not identical, concerns. Given their own work ethic, counselors took pride in their agency, which did not operate a "giveaway" program, but were perplexed by those who only wanted a handout. Goals were an undeniable, if not altogether desirable, feature of their agency. Consequently, the counselors were somewhat ambivalent about their agency's recent shift in policy. Desiring to serve people, they welcomed the emphasis on substantial services. Yet working in an agency that continued to stress production, they were concerned that the shift in policy might make "getting their numbers" more difficult. Within these organizational and professional concerns, the rehabilitation counselors served clients. To do so, counselors worked cases.

NOTES

1. Official publications of the state agency and other public sources have been used in this discussion. However, they are not cited because to do so would destroy the agency's anonymity.

2. These figures vary from year to year. They are a rough indication of the cost-effectiveness of rehabilitation. They are not as precise as the benefit-cost ratios discussed in the previous chapter. The figure cited here does not take into account the funds spent on clients who were not rehabilitated. Nor does it take into account (estimated) changes in employment (for better or for worse) during an individual's employment history. It does not reflect the extra taxes the rehabilitated clients will be paying or the decrease in public support payments and institutional care.

3. Other counselors who worked for the state vocational rehabilitation department were located in state facilities, such as a mental health hospital or a facility for the mentally retarded. Their work would be slightly different from the field counselor's. The bulk of public vocational rehabilitation counselors are field counselors. Approximately 80 percent were in the state where I observed.

4. However, area offices and their supervisors were not as autonomous as were the branch offices and their supervisors in a midwestern parole agency (McCleary, 1978: 50-60).

5. During the course of my research the position of quality control specialist was retitled "counselor 3" ("3" to designate third level), though the duties did not change.

6. Similar reviews of (intended) services and courses of action are undertaken in other human service agencies (Buckholdt and Gubrium, 1979a: chap. 5; Gubrium and Buckholdt, 1982: chap. 5).

7. Typically, counselors had their own casework assistants, which, according to a state administrator, was a departure from other states' practices where pools of secretaries provided typing and other services.

8. See Murphy and Ursprung (1983) for a discussion of how vocational evaluations were conducted in two different vocational evaluation facilities. They found that evaluations were not merely a result of clinical judgments, but also grew out of the evaluators'"awareness of consequences of their analysis for the career of the client and for subsequent actions of the professional community" (Murphy and Ursprung, 1983: 2).

9. Prottas (1979: 245) argues that the waiting area and the need to wait demeaned welfare clients in the welfare department he observed. In contrast, the rehabilitation clients waited in relatively pleasant, uncrowded surroundings. However, once informed that a client or potential client was waiting to see him or her, a counselor did not

immediately drop what he or she was doing to see the individual. Paperwork or a cup of coffee might be finished within a few minutes before the individual was seen.

10. Counselors did not specialize according to the various functions of the rehabilitation process, such as case finding or job placement. One state administrator noted that with placement specialists

> the counselor has a little less ownership [of the case], and we think . . . if a counselor from day one, when he is interviewing a client, is thinking placement, thinking going back to work, thinking job, then he will have more ownership in and do a little better job.

See Wright (1980: 59-66) for a discussion about specialization.

11. According to a state administrator, goals for successful closures were based on the estimated number of placement possibilities in a year divided by the number of counselors. The estimated number of placement possibilites was based on 10 percent of the number of jobs that the state's Employment Security Commission estimated would be filled during the year (10 percent because approximately 10 percent of the jobs in the state were held by disabled individuals) adjusted for the closures expected to be homemakers and those working for their families, which would not be listed with the employment commission. Goals for successful closures varied by the nature of the caseload, by the experience of the counselor, and by the region of the state (goals for the counselors in the area office I observed were slightly higher than elsewhere). The goals for plans were set approximately 10 to 20 plans more than "26s" because some plans ended in unsuccessful closures.

12. This counselor's emphasis on the importance of work is echoed by other rehabilitation professionals:

> Despite criticism of its narrow focus, experience with vocational rehabilitation indicates that other problem areas [for example, family] may not require outside intervention if the disabled person can be returned to work [Wright, 1980: 77].

13. The general guideline for the number of active cases (that is, those in which a plan had been developed) was 125 plus or minus 10. However, according to one official, 125 was too high. The official noted that many successful counselors had active caseloads of 90 to 95, which allowed them to "concentrate their efforts, . . . do a better job, and therefore get a faster turn[over]."

14. Caseload size itself may not be as detrimental to the quality of the cases' outcomes as counselors' complaints suggest (Zadny and James, 1979a). The same is true in other human service agencies, such as parole and probation departments (Empey, 1978: 508-510). While large caseload size may not be as detrimental to service as commonly imagined, "marginal" reductions in size ("say, from 50 to 45 cases") may not be as effective as hoped for but could be quite expensive if demand were to remain the same (Lispky, 1980: 205-236).

15. A survey of M.A.-level rehabilitation students three years after they graduated indicated that relatively few felt concerned about their agency's "pressure for results" (Sussman and Haug, 1970).

3

WORKING CASES

To do their job, detectives work cases. Law enforcement detectives "gather, organize, and use information about social behavior" in order to solve crimes (Sanders, 1977: 12). To do so, they attempt to establish cases, identify and locate suspects, "cop the suspects" (that is, obtain a confession from them), and then dispose of the cases (Sanders, 1977: 79). If detectives are successful, then crimes have been solved; cases have been cleared. To serve clients, rehabilitation counselors and other human service professionals work cases, too.

In order to serve individuals with vocationally handicapping disabilities, rehabilitation counselors work cases. By developing, organizing, and using information, counselors attempt to establish that individuals are eligible for the agency's services, to "make a case" for the individuals. If done successfully, individuals then become clients. Transforming individuals into clients is a fundamental task for rehabilitation and other human service detectives (Euler, 1979; Prottas, 1979). If cases are not made, then there are no clients to serve, and how cases are made influences how clients are served. Once cases are made, plans of services are enacted and the cases are managed to their conclusion. In this chapter, I examine how rehabilitation counselors worked cases from their initial contact with potential clients through the development of plans of services and how they attempted to make cases and dealt with their inability to do so. In the following chapter, I will explain how counselors managed cases from the development of a plan of services to their conclusion—how they concluded cases. These counselors worked cases—both making and concluding them—within an agency that had a profound impact on how cases were worked. If there seemed to be contradictions and inconsistencies in the collective and the individual working of cases, then perhaps it was due to the contradictions and inconsistencies that appeared sometimes within and among the agency's, counselors', *and* clients' concerns.

In working cases, counselors established initially whether or not an individual referred to them should be evaluated. If counselors decided to *open a case,* then typically they gathered information to *make a case* for the applicant. If a case was successfully made, then a *plan* of services was developed. However, some applicants were established to be ineligible for services, and others did not participate sufficiently during the investigation for their eligibility to be established. The former's disappointment was managed by *cooling them out,* and the latter's lack of meaningful involvement was documented by *making a case against them.* Thus in working cases, counselors handled both those that might later become successful closures after having been made and those that were closed without even having been made.

OPENING A CASE

In order to work cases, rehabilitation counselors must have cases to work. While detectives (with the general exception of vice and narcotic detectives) typically depend on the reports of patrol officers to bring crimes to their attention, counselors encourage community agencies and individuals to bring potential clients to their attention. Detectives are *reactive.* They react to the field reports of patrol officers, who have themselves typically reacted to the complaints of citizens. Rehabilitation counselors are much more *proactive.* They seek out potential cases to work by developing and working referral sources, which is one of the key tasks in managing their caseloads (see Chapter 5).

Counselors developed and worked referral sources not only to obtain cases to work, but also to control the kinds of cases they obtained. However, some referrals turned out not to be cases at all, and some cases were better than others. As I explain later, "good" cases (a term that had various meanings, depending on organizational and counselors' concerns) were desired, though certainly not always obtained. Counselors further controlled their work by deciding whether or not to open a case on individuals referred to them.

Counselors, like other human service professionals (Prottas, 1979: 30-31; Peyrot, 1982), did not open a case (take an application) on all the referred individuals they saw.[1] They did not even see all the individuals referred to them. Counselors were expected to screen out those who were "clearly" inappropriate or ineligible and were criticized for being "afraid to say no." Several counselors remarked that they had become, or needed to and intended to become, more selective in opening cases on referrals. But who was screened out, and how was this done?

Unlike detectives, who are made aware of crimes through the reports of patrol officers, rehabilitation counselors became aware of referrals through various kinds of reports and, more frequently, through encounters with the individuals, either over the telephone or in person. Counselors received "paper referrals," such as transmittals from their Disability Determination Division, which reported that individuals had received, been denied, or terminated social security benefits. Or, counselors who worked public school caseloads distributed a "physical condition survey" to students to generate referrals. Counselors screened these and other kinds of paper referrals before attempting to contact some of the individuals. For those seen in person, whether preceded by a paper referral or not, counselors interviewed the referrals to determine whether or not a case should be opened.[2]

While there was variation among counselors as to whom they screened out, counselors usually attempted to screen out the following: those few referrals who indicated no significant physical, mental, or emotional disability; those who only wanted the agency to buy them something; and those who were not interested in returning to work (or working with the counselor) or for whom it was extremely doubtful they could return to work. When paper referrals were screened, counselors attended to the first and third categories of "undesirables," and, when encountering referrals in person, all three categories became relevant. Counselors who opened a case on "anyone" because all who sought services were legally entitled to an evaluation or counselors who were "crusaders"—who "thought it was [their] job in a sense to yank everybody in here that had some sort of handicap"—often experienced difficulty later in working the cases (Euler, 1979: 55).

Paper Referrals

When screening paper referrals, counselors faced the task of determining whether or not to contact the individuals personally. In making that decision, counselors assessed whether the referral seemed to have a "significant" disability that might provide the basis for the agency's involvement or whether the referral's situation seemed so unpromising that successful involvement was unlikely. Within the context of meeting their goals, the counselors made those decisions based on experience, practical reasoning, and their personal orientations to their work.[3]

For example, when counselors who worked public school caseloads received unmarked "physical condition survey" forms from students, the counselors did not contact the students. Those paper referrals were screened out. Counselors might also screen out, or contact much later in the year, those students who checked such conditions as "become tired very easily," "sinuses (painful, draining, infected)," and/or "severe headaches." Based on experience, some counselors learned that such referrals rarely became cases. After questioning the students, the counselors found that the "severe headaches," "sinuses," and "become tired very easily" often turned out to be infrequent, mundane occurrences that students claimed were causing them no significant difficulty. One counselor reasoned that if such conditions were significant, then the students would eventually be referred to the counselor through some other means. However, another, reasoning that it took only a few minutes to question the students, might promptly request that the students see him. Unrecognized problems might even be uncovered. However, such reasoning was not used by counselors as a justification for contacting students who had not checked any condition.

When screening paper referrals, counselors also assessed whether or not the referral's situation seemed so unpromising that successful involvement was very unlikely. With paper referrals this concern primarily arose when counselors received transmittals from the Disability Determination Division, particularly those indicating that individuals had been denied social security disability benefits. Counselors generally viewed "DDD denials" as unpromising possibilities. The individuals often had severe disabilities, but, perhaps more important, they had claimed they could not work and were often resentful that their claims had been denied. Some might "use" the agency in order to receive additional medical evaluations to be used in an appeal. Others, appealing their decision, had no interest in being involved in the agency. As one counselor remarked of DDD denials,

A lot of counselors I think kind of shy away from using those because they are severe, very severe. They are people who have said, "I can never work," and they have been turned down, and so you have a few marks against you.

While counselors viewed DDD denials as unpromising, that view depended, in part, on the quality of referrals received routinely elsewhere. After being transferred from a caseload that had a reliable, predictable flow of cases that were "guaranteed to be eligible" to a general caseload requiring more digging for cases, one counselor began to rely more heavily on DDD denials. On the other hand, what was unpromising to other counselors might be viewed as "at least worth a contact" to the counselor who handled cases involving disability beneficiaries. Thus one general counselor noted that if a DDD denial involved a 50-year-old who last worked 10 or 15 years ago, then the woman would not be interested in working and would not be contacted. Yet a counselor who served disability beneficiaries (and, until special federal funds were no longer appropriated, worked under different guidelines than fellow counselors) decided to contact a 39-year-old woman with a ninth-grade education and no work history but with multiple disabilities—schizophrenia, seizures, and high blook pressure. While the referral did not look "good," the recipient's condition was to be reviewed by the Social Security Administration in approximately one year, at which time the counselor felt the recipient would "probably" be cut off due to stricter eligibility decisions that had recently become effective. While the beneficiary might or might not cooperate with the counselor, the counselor felt that individual needed the agency's services. Thus what was unpromising to counselors was a relative matter, relative to the kinds of cases with which counselors typically worked.

When counselors did not screen out paper referrals, the interview became the key to whether counselors opened a case or not. As one counselor remarked, "So, you never know until they come in and you have a personal interview with them."[4] The same sentiments applied to those referrals who were initially seen in person.

The Interview

Interviews are crucial in detective work. In working cases, detectives may question victims, witnesses, knowledgeable persons, and (possible) suspects. Through interviews, detectives gather much of the information needed to solve cases. Interviews are crucial, too, for rehabilitation and human service detectives (McCleary, 1978; Prottas, 1979; Lipsky, 1980: 120-122).[5]

Rehabilitation professionals emphasized the importance of the initial interview with the referral (Britten, 1981). A quality control specialist remarked to new counselors who were studying the agency's case manual that counselors never felt the same about cases that had been transferred to them as they did about those for which they had conducted the initial interview. Initial interviews were also important because they might have been the longest single contact between counselors and clients. The same seems to be true for other human service detectives, such as intake workers in welfare agencies (Prottas, 1979: 26). However, the length of interviews varied greatly. I witnessed initial interviews that lasted from fifteen minutes to an hour and a half and heard of some that went on longer.[6]

Initial interviews were especially important because of what counselors were attemping to accomplish in that meeting. First, counselors tried to decide whether or not further investigation was needed. If a case was opened, then the counselor attempted to establish a working relationship with the applicant that would aid in the case's successful making and closure.[7]

SCREENING REFERRALS

Due to their development and working of referral sources and their screening of paper referrals, counselors interviewed relatively few referrals who obviously lacked some kind of significant disability. Some "walk-ins" (people who walked in from the streets without an appointment and without being referred) might be deemed inappropriate. One counselor explained:

> The walk-in people sometimes are that. They walk in and just—they reach you and then they are not sure who they are reaching for. Sometimes I have spent a couple of hours with people who really didn't need us. And one lady who came to me, I found out after it was all over. She got real upset. She was applying for a job as a janitor. She said, "Why you keep talking about disability?" . . . Somehow she thought she was up there applying for a job as a janitor.

Counselors who worked school caseloads occasionally saw students who, upon extensive questioning, reported no disability that appeared to be a potentially significant obstacle to employment. As I noted earlier, these counselors typically used a physical condition survey as one means of generating referrals. After screening these paper referrals, counselors contacted some of the students and subsequently determined that some did not have any problems that needed the agency's attention. Students who reported sinus problems, skin allergies, emotional problems, sore knees and headaches, vision problems, or ulcers might be contacted, but when the counselors learned that the medical conditions were under control, had cleared up, were not felt to be important to the student, or were not causing the student any problems, then counselors did not investigate the cases further. Such referrals agreed with the counselors' observation that they did not need vocational rehabilitation services.

Counselors also attempted to screen out referrals who were not interested in returning to work, including those who only wanted the agency to buy them something—medication, medical evaluation, glasses, and the like. Referrals who clearly stated that they had no intention of returning to work posed no problem for the counselors. However, the intentions of other referrals were not so clear to the counselors, and perhaps not even to the referrals themselves. Counselors, however, did not begin an interview with the intention of screening out the current referral for not intending to work. Instead, counselors were aware of the possibility that some referrals had no intention of returning to work and, during the course of the interview, may have suspected that the referral was uninterested in working.[8] Additionally, any citizen who wanted an evaluation to determine eligibility was entitled to one. Therefore, counselors tended to manage the encounters with referrals so that referrals screened themselves out. To varying degrees they did so in three ways.

Counselors asked referrals directly, sometimes repeatedly, and, in a few instances I witnessed, with an almost inquisitorial tone, whether or not they wanted to return to work. Counselors also emphasized to the referrals the work orientation of their agency. They stressed that their agency was not a "giveaway" program. Instead, they explained, by becoming successfully employed, referrals enabled counselors to serve future clients because the agency's funding was based on the successful rehabilitation of individuals. At times counselors seemed to be trying to develop an almost moral obligation on the referral's part to follow through, an obligation emphasized by other human service professionals too, such as Work Incentive Program counselors (Miller, 1983). Finally, the individual was told that if the counselor was to help the referral become successfully rehabilitated, much would be expected of the referral: appointments kept, evaluations undertaken, counseling sessions attended, jobs sought, and so forth. After being told what their responsibility would be in their own rehabilitation, some referrals decided it would be too much responsibility and did not ask that a case be opened.[9] As one counselor explained:

> Sometimes I'll sit down and go over with them, "Now you know you're going to have to keep all your appointments with me, and I'm going to see you at least on a bi-monthly basis, and we're going to be sending you out for employer interviews, and we're going to be expecting you to keep— we're going to be setting you up for job club meetings so that we can . . . fill out the job applications and go through interview techniques." And sometimes, you know, once they realize exactly what their end of the bargain's gonna be and what they're going to be expected to maintain, they realize that that's a little more than they bargained for.

Counselors also screened out cases in which they believed it was extremely doubtful the referred individuals would return to work. As one counselor explained:

> I was referred . . . a gentleman who was a chronic alcoholic, going blind from diabetic retinopathy—severe visual problems from diabetic retinopathy with severe pancreatitis. I talked with the guy a few minutes and pretty much decided I did not think he was feasible for VR services. Other things entered into it. First, the guy had no address. His only address right now was the [name] Hospital. He had been sleeping in his car prior to admission to the hospital. I did not feel he was a good risk, a good candidate for services, so I told them, "No thank you."

However, counselors opened cases when referrals "really wanted their help" or "wanted to work," even if the counselors felt that the likelihood of the referrals' returning to work was small. As one counselor remarked:

> I have clients that, for example, my professional opinion was that they were too severe, but I took the case anyway. If they told me they really wanted my help. I can think of one right now . . . where I honestly believed

then and I still believe that his prognosis is about zero, I mean, how much is it going to hurt me to try?

That counselor felt that his orientation was the exception, but I disagree. Another counselor noted:

What I'm trying to tell you is if somebody says they want some services, I'm willing to give it a shot. You know, I guess the background at [name] Hospital [where the counselor once worked]. You lose so many people and you have so many frustrations going over and over again . . . but, you know, if you try a lot, the more you try, the more chances of success.

Counselors' sentiments regarding referrals who had "good attitudes" but problematic chances of successful rehabilitation must be understood in the context of organizational and counselors' concerns. Referrals who were seen in person and who had "good attitudes" struck a sympathetic note with counselors concerned with serving people. Whether counselors opened a case or directed the referrals to another part of their agency (for example, to a program in independent living) or to another agency, they were responding from a desire to provide service. If later in the rehabilitation process evaluation revealed no potential or no significant progress was made, counselors then responded to the need to meet their goals. Correspondingly, counselors did not seek "hopeless" cases. In the faceless screening of paper referrals, counselors screened out those they felt had poor potential for returning to work. Counselors responded to two concerns, which was not always easy to do or always consistently done.

By deciding whether or not to open a case, counselors attempted to increase control over their work (and with whom they worked) and the likelihood of obtaining successful closures. They were only partially successful. As in other agencies, control is never complete and uncertainty is never eliminated (Gubrium and Buckholdt, 1982: 131). While relatively few cases were opened in which counselors later decided the applicants were not eligible for services, through lack of cooperation, refusal of services, or inability to remain in contact with the counselors, many more applicants' cases were closed without a case having been made for them.[10] Some of these applicants had little motivation to work, but indicated they would try and that they were interested in the agency's program. As one counselor noted of such applicants:

They say, "Maybe I could go to work if you got me where I was feeling better and you could find the right job where on the days I don't feel like going in I wouldn't have to go in, you know . . . " and they say, "Well, some days I just don't even feel like getting out of bed. If you could find me a job where the employer would understand that, I might would go to work." Well, you don't have a whole lot of choice. They understand what the services are. They have disability. It's keeping them from work. And they are telling you that they are willing to give it a shot at going to work. You got to open a case.

Some had probably "conned" the counselors, and others might not have completely appreciated what was expected of them or later decided not to do what counselors expected them to do. Once counselors realized that these cases were going nowhere, they tried to close them ("08") so they could deal with more promising cases. How they did so is discussed later in the chapter.

ESTABLISHING A WORKING RELATIONSHIP

When counselors opened a case, they attempted to establish a working relationship with the applicants. Counselors further worked the cases based on the initial relationship created. Much of what counselors did in their attempts to screen out inappropriate referrals also served to establish a working relationship.

Counselors informed applicants of what the agency did, the kinds of services that were offered and might be provided to the applicants (that is, "selling" the agency to the applicants; Willey, 1979), their responsibility in rehabilitation, and what the next steps in the process would be. Some counselors began to advise applicants regarding job-seeking skills and job possibilities. In a few cases, counselors worked themselves out of a case because such advice enabled the applicants to find employment. Consequently, the applicants were no longer interested in and/or eligible for the agency's services. Thus counselors attempted to educate the applicants and elicit their future cooperation, a task also faced by law enforcement detectives and other human service professionals (Prottas, 1979: 78; Lipsky, 1980: 61-65; Sanders, 1980: 91-94).

When counselors questioned the referrals, they also developed an initial understanding of the cases and how they would work them. Counselors questioned the referrals about their "problems"—their nature, duration, perceived limitations, impact on work, treatment sought, and so forth—and what the referrals wanted from the agency. The counselors attempted to develop information and strategies that could be used in making a case for the applicants (such as establishing their eligibility) and later successfully concluding the case (that is, successfully rehabilitating the clients). For example, if a referral mentioned that he or she had little self-confidence or many family problems, or if he or she had a low score on an IQ test, then the counselor might tentatively plan for a basic psychological evaluation to be conducted. If a referral complained of continuing headaches that interfered with school or work, then the counselor mentally noted that a neurological exam might be in order. If a referral mentioned employment possibilities the counselors felt would be difficult to achieve due to the referral's capabilities or because the jobs would not be readily available in the area, then the counselor might urge the referral to be more realistic. For example, when one referral expressed an interest in portrait photography, the counselor questioned the referral as to whether he thought employment possibilities in the community in that field were good or not. The counselor told the referral, who had not thought about the job market, that freelance photographers often did not earn a good living. Other counselors might wait until later in the investigative work to encourage an applicant to be more realistic. At the interview stage, anything was a possibility. In developing a working relationship with the applicant and the case, a counselor was usually beginning to make a case as well.

One counselor explained about initial interviews:

> What I try to do in my initial interview is to determine what's going on, who's involved, what's happening, what type of . . . job that might interest her [speaking of a female applicant], what are her job responsibilities [the applicant is currently working], and what she feels like, or what she wants to do about it if anything. Also, looking for any signs of information or signs that I can detect as a counselor that will aid in: (1) either establishing eligibility; (2) bring out the alleged disability or such like that.

When counselors opened a case, they concluded the interviews with the referrals by completing the application. They used the application as a tool to elicit information to develop a working relationship, as well as to record the information received. Some counselors centered the interview on the application; others completed it after more extensive questioning of the referrals. Counselors were urged by the QCs and the area supervisor to fill in the application completely, with particular emphasis on obtaining good references and directions to the applicant's home. Those two pieces of information could be useful in contacting applicants (and, later, clients) who did not keep in touch.

After the application was completed, the counselors had the applicants sign release forms that enabled the counselors to obtain information concerning the applicants from other agencies, such as schools or hospitals. Counselors quickly conducted an "analysis of economic circumstances" to determine if the applicants were eligible for "cost" services—any planned services purchased by the agency, such as surgery, prostheses, psychotherapy, or training. The applicants' eligibility for cost services was not usually a problem for the counselors because either the applicants obviously met the economic requirements (they were unemployed) or no cost services were likely to be provided. Finally, counselors usually gave applicants a General Medical Examination Report form and asked them to thave it filled out as soon as possible by their doctor (at the agency's expense) or referred them to a doctor who accepted the agency's applicants and clients (and fees). The cases were open; now they needed to be made.

MAKING A CASE

Once counselors opened a case, they attempted to make a case—in other words, to establish the applicant's eligibility for the agency's services. To do so, they needed to document that the applicant had met two criteria:

(1) the presence of a physical or mental disability that for the individual constitutes or results in a substantial handicap to employment
(2) a reasonable expectation that vocational rehabilitation services may benefit the individual in terms of employability

Counselors viewed the establishment of an applicant's eligibility as self-evident. While evidence had to be gathered to document the applicant's eligibility, this task was seen as routine. According to one counselor, it was not difficult to decide if an applicant was eligible or not. However, such routine cases masked a fundamental feature of establishing eligibility: Counselors always *made* applicants eligible. I do not mean that counselors "made up" the applicant's eligibility, though they and other rehabilitation professionals did comment on the sometimes not-so-appropriate actions of fellow counselors. For example, counselors were "fussed at" for trying to make an applicant eligible for dental work. Or, as one counselor noted:

> The key [to writing a plan] first of all is having somebody that's eligible, not "making somebody eligible," have somebody who is eligible. . . . I just tell you that people don't have problems with quality control if what they're doing is legitimate. The thing is, that's when they try to say, "Well, what if I said this?" as if, you know, we're wheeling-dealing in a back room. Dammit, just be right, you know. You have a client. What is in the best interest of that client? Is that person eligible? I cannot believe that an eligible person is going to get turned down. I just don't believe it.

However, eligibility did not reside within the clients' makeup. Eligibility did not exist apart from a counselor's investigative work and documentation. Routine cases obscured that fact. In many cases, any competent counselor would engage in similar activities and reach similar outcomes. Eligibility or ineligibility seemed to be independent of the counselor's activities. These activities were taken for granted and had become largely routinized. Such routinization enabled counselors to do their work in a professional, orderly manner that reduced the inherent uncertainty in any investigative process and obscured for rehabilitation professionals and outside observers the complete dependence of applicants' eligibility on the work of counselors. The work involved became more visible in problematic cases in which counselors were not sure how to proceed or others questioned how they had proceeded. Many times in case development staffings (see Chapter 5) counselors asked their fellow counselors and QCs if they had "enough to write a plan," or "is this an 08 or a plan" or asked what they should do next. Discussion would sometimes be extensive, as the following *condensed* exchange indicates:

Supervisor: Any more plans?

Counselor 1: Yeah, uh, this is a homemaker. Real bad, out-of-control blood pressure with the usual things you find with it. I guess you'd say dizziness and getting weak . . . Oh, she had a complaint with her eyes, too. We sent her for a checkup on her eyes because her eyes did look like they had a wide gaze. Dr. [name] recommended we do muscle surgery, no glasses needed. Her vision really is not bad. In fact, her vision for close is normal and the distance is just a slight loss. Anyway, he didn't recommend anything but that. But Dr. [medical consultant's name] looked at it and says that there is no bearing on her ability to do homemaking or anything else with this visual thing. Her vision is okay. So this would just be for appearance. So we don't see that. But the blood pressure on general medical was 170/115 to give you some idea of how poor the control can be with her blood pressure. And Dr. [name] worked her up and said that it was poorly controlled and recommended that we provide some follow-up to control her blood pressure so I was going to propose, there again, several visits to the doctor for control of her blood pressure.

Supervisor: The question I have on that case is what are *we* going to do? What do you plan to do? What kind of direct service are we going to deliver from a vocational rehabilitation standpoint?

Counselor 1: Well, with someone like that who doesn't know anything about her work tolerance, when it would be right to return to work or return to her activities, I think we could fill that gap . . .

Supervisor: It seems to me that that would be a case where really all we are doing is paying a bill and not really getting involved with any direct service ourselves. How do ya'll see it? What do ya'll think [name of second counselor]?

Counselor 2: How exactly is the blood pressure interfering with her homemaking duties?

Counselor 1: Dizziness, being tired a lot, that kind of thing.

Counselor 2: Is she performing any of them now?

Counselor 1: Yeah, she's performing some. She's not able to do it to the extent that it really needs to be done. She's got three children that try to do it all for her.

Supervisor: I'm not, I wouldn't question whether or not she needs treatment for hypertension. It's obvious that she does. I think with our new guidelines . . . that we do have to deliver a direct service to those clients. I think we need to be real clear what we are going to deliver. The only thing that I could really hang my hat on from what you said is the treatment for the hypertension. The lady is not retarded or anything like that, so, therefore, she should know when to take her medication and that kind of thing. [name of second counselor], help us . . .

Counselor 2: You don't believe she would cooperate with trying to come over here for any formal adjustment services or even a regular counseling type of thing about dealing with those problems. [supervisor's name], would that justify it?

Supervisor: I think you would have a problem justifying it like that unless the lady was emotionally, had some kind of anxiety reaction to this . . .

Counselor 1: She probably wouldn't be able to leave the home anyway with a family. She's got three children to supervise in the mornings and afternoons and all that too. So she's not a candidate for coming to [city] for a workshop or anything of that kind.

Supervisor: All our services would be directed toward the disability and not towards the vocational objective.

Counselor 1: Um hum. It would be toward stabilizing her realistically rather than have her just get some prescriptions again and maybe do what's been done in the past.

Counselor 2: There's one thing in here [case folder]. It says she is obese. How obese is she? Wait a minute it says 5'5", 250 pounds.

Supervisor: Whew! . . .

Counselor 2: Could this not be something that counseling is needed for? Or, if she could get in here, I know [the adjustment specialist] works with that in the adjustment courses.

Counselor 1: Like I said, I don't see this woman leaving her family to come to a workshop, but we can ask her.

Supervisor: Does the client see this as a problem, the obesity as a problem, or how would she react to that?

Counselor 1: Hadn't mentioned it. I was told by the people in the state office very clearly that we didn't write plans for treatment or for affecting anything in reference to losing weight. That they did not buy it as a realistic maneuver.

Supervisor: That's certainly true. I would agree with that wholeheartedly, but obviously her obesity is affecting the hypertension. It's the hypertension that is the problem, but if she lost weight, she may be able to control the hypertension better.

Counselor 1: So you see a potential service if this lady is interested in getting active to come to the workshop to work on her.

Supervisor: If we could offer her adjustment services to work on her obesity and maybe her work stamina and being able to take care of some specific homemaking duties that she can't do now, then I think we might have a solid case there.

Counselor 1: Okay, let's see what she says about that.

Supervisor: Do ya'll agree with that? And our direct service in that would be what in your opinion, [Counselor 2]?

Counselor 2: Counseling with her on taking the medication, on the permanence of the condition, on the obesity, on how it all interacts, and on the issue that taking one pill a day is not going to solve the problem . . .

Supervisor: First thing, [Counselor 1], see if she can come in for some personal, social adjustment three times a week or whatever you can work out with her. If she can't do that, then let's go that route like [Counselor 2] is saying, let's write it up and go ahead and write the plan up emphasizing that your counseling would be directed toward weight control, taking the medication, explaining to her how it all relates together with the hypertension and obesity together and the problems that that causes, and let's see what we can do. That sounds like a better service and how this relates to her not being able to perform her homemaking duties.

Counselor 2: One of the goals being to increase the work tolerance, and you need the counseling on the obesity for that.

Supervisor: Yeah. Maybe getting her on some kind of exercise program at home or something like that.

Counselor 1: The reason I discounted that was, like I said, I had thought that they wouldn't, the quality control would not pass on anything when you get into weight loss.

Supervisor: As a primary disability, you're just about right. . . . I think they came out with a chart one time, but, God, you have to be, crazy kinds of stuff, you have to be 900 pounds overweight. . . . Where you have a medical diagnosis that obviously the obesity is causing some problems in contributing toward that problem, the medical problem, then certainly we can counsel about the obesity and how it relates to the medical problem, building her work stamina, and how it relates to not being able to do some homemaking duties. So you might be able to hang your hat on that.

Counselor 1: Sounds good to me. I just didn't think we could write it that way.

Counselor 2: Low-salt diet.

Supervisor: Low-salt diet, those kinds of things. Giving her some information on proper diet. And maybe [the adjustment specialist] could help you with getting some information on it.

Problematic cases such as the above also distorted what took place. Such cases gave the impression that all was uncertainty in rehabilitation work, when in fact it was not. Rehabilitation work was a mixture of uncertainty and routine. Yet in all cases, counselors had to make the case for the applicant. The same is true in any human service agency (Prottas, 1979; Lipsky, 1980: 59-70).

In order to make a case, counselors had to establish the four elements of eligibility: *disability, vocational handicap, services,* and *vocational objective.* The counselors needed to demonstrate their interrelationship and compatibility. The disability produced "functional limitations" that were a substantial handicap to employment. The planned services must, in the words of one QC, "remove, reduce, or work around" that which was causing the functional limitations. Finally, those services must have a "reasonable" possibility of enabling the applicant to be employed successfully in a position compatible with the applicants' capabilities and remaining disabilities. And in making a case, counselors dealt with applicants whose own concerns and desires might pose problems of accommodation.

The Disability: Establishing an "Angle"

Counselors needed to establish that applicants had a diagnosed disability in order for them to be eligible for services. In doing so, counselors tried to establish an "angle." By "angle" counselors meant more than the applicant's disability, though typically the disability was the initial and most important feature of an angle. By analogy, a reporter, being a different kind of detective, develops an angle for a story—a framework or focus for the event to be reported (Altheide, 1976: 73-83). Detectives, too, construct angles when they establish that a reported incident is a certain kind of crime (for example, a reported case of attempted murder is established to be really a "glorified domestic"; Sanders, 1977: 84-99).

Establishing a disability was generally routine. An up-to-date diagnosis from a doctor or a psychologist was sufficient. A general medical evaluation (or its equivalent, such as a recent hospital examination), which was required of all applicants, specialty exams, and psychological evaluations generally provided the needed diagnosis. The applicant's "presenting" problem was supported. But not always:

> Being a released inmate from another state, the applicant was psychologically evaluated by the staff psychologist. [Offenders typically became eligible based on psychological disabilities.] The evaluation revealed no significant disability. The counselor then arranged for a neurosurgeon to examine the applicant, who had been complaining of lower back pain. Nothing significant was found. A neurologist then examined the applicant, and an EMG was performed, which again showed nothing. After the medical consultant reviewed the findings, the case was closed "08," no disabling condition.

Without a disability, counselors did not have a case. Therefore (as the above case indicates), they might be advised to try or they might try other angles on their own if the initial angles did not work out. They might go the "psychological route" for applicants who complained of "blanking out" though no visual problems existed, those who were overweight but without physical complications, those who complained of headaches but for whom neither a general medical evaluation nor a neurological exam showed anything, or those who, as students, came in "for a dental."

In establishing a disability, counselors might test and retest the applicants. This occurred with applicants when the angle was mental retardation. Applicants who scored above, but near, the agency cutoff of 75 on an IQ test might be retested in the hope they would score 75 or below. Without a score of 75 or below, an applicant could not be diagnosed as mentally retarded, though such a test score was not sufficient by itself. Applicants must also have had functional limitations that pointed to their difficulty in working. However, one QC noted that the "state people" would look closely if many IQ tests were given. Yet a counselor argued that the agency should be able to serve someone with an "IQ score of 76 and who was in special education classes in school." The test was a fallible tool for assessing an applicant's abilities and disabilities. This concern with the use of tests and evaluations to establish eligibility was expressed in one staffing by a counselor who joked that an applicant who apparently had no significant disability should be "tested in a wind tunnel" in order to find something wrong.

If tests were fallible, then so too were the staff psychologist and medical consultant. Counselors approached them with the intention of having them support the case they were building. As one counselor remarked of the staff psychologist:

> You're looking for him to be the one to give you a diagnosis or concur with the diagnosis you have so you can proceed with services. You very seldom go to him to rule out and say, "make this person ineligible," you know, or something like that.

However, the psychologist or the consultant might not support the counselors' angles, either asking for additional medical information or failing to provide the desired diagnosis.[11] If that happened, then counselors might try to work around the consultants, perhaps staffing the case with the QC so additional information need not be sought, or looking elsewhere for needed information. For example, if the staff psychologist did not give a disability on an applicant, then a counselor might try to convince the applicant to go to a local area mental health center in order to obtain a diagnosis that would enable the counselor to work with the applicant. However, as one counselor noted, counselors would have their hands slapped if they went "over the head" of the psychologist too often.

The counselors' practices of trying different angles or going to great lengths to "get a diagnosis" should not be understood as illegitimate. Instead, those practices are best understood within organizational and counselors' concerns. The case manual advised counselors that

> insofar as possible, every opportunity should be taken to serve clients rather than reject them. Every effort should be made to explore possibilities thoroughly in order to find appropriate avenues for providing services.

While making "every effort" was an impossible requirement, in trying to get a diagnosis, counselors were attempting to serve people and to meet their goals.

Substantiating a Vocational Handicap

Once counselors obtained a diagnosed disability, they had to establish that it was a substantial handicap to employment.[12] "Disability" and "vocational handicap" were not synonymous. For example, one QC told counselors repeatedly that when an applicant scored below 75 on an IQ test it did not make that person automatically eligible for the agency's services. Counselors must also document functional limitations—such as an inability to follow directions, count money, or take public transportation—that would interfere with employment. *Controlled* diabetes or hypertension did not constitute a substantial vocational handicap. The following incident from a case development staffing indicates the difference between a disability and a vocational handicap (as well as how the failure to establish that the former constitutes the latter may lead to the reworking of a case):

> A counselor staffed for plan a case of a young woman who was cross-eyed, but who also had a "little minor heart condition," "some kind of valve disorder." The counselor intended to provide counseling, guidance, and placement assistance in a food service or housekeeper position. Given the

client's heart condition, others questioned the vocational objective of housekeeper. The counselor responded that the client's valve disorder had not "prevented her from living a normal, active life." Upon hearing that, the QC remarked that the heart condition was not a vocational handicap. After a brief discussion, the counselor decided to get a "psychological" and "check the eyes."

Counselors must establish that the disability made a vocational difference. They did so in various ways. Applicants who lost their jobs or whose jobs were in jeopardy (as noted by the applicants' supervisors) because of the impairments were assumed to have vocational handicaps, and it was so documented. The general medical exam and the specialty exams might provide information about the disability's impact on the applicant's work. If not, or if the reports were not clear to the counselors, then the medical and psychological consultants would be asked to provide such information. School officials and reports often provided useful information concerning the functional limitations (difficulties) of student applicants. During the initial interviews with referrals, counselors often elicited problems the referrals were having or had on their previous jobs. Evaluation at the rehabilitation center often provided the needed information. Perhaps most important, a substantial handicap was established by showing that the agency could provide substantial services to the applicant. If the agency could become substantially involved with the applicant, then the applicant must have a substantial handicap. The former became proof of the latter.

Substantial Services: "What Are We Going to Do?"

In order to make a case, counselors needed to show that through the agency and/or its sponsorship, substantial services could appropriately be provided to the applicant. As stated in the agency's manual:

Services provided by this agency and its agents must be above and beyond those already available to all persons and not otherwise obtainable from other resources.

As a practical concern, counselors needed to establish, to the satisfaction of quality control specialists, that what they were planning to do made a difference and was not simply paying a bill. As I noted in the previous chapter, any time the counselors could show the need for counseling and guidance and job placement, they were showing a need for substantial services. Typically that was a routine matter, especially for applicants without jobs (but not always, as indicated by the lengthy excerpt presented earlier from a case development staffing that concerned the problems of establishing eligibility). Often it was assumed to be obvious that applicants who were mentally retarded, suffered from drug abuse, or had mental health or emotional problems needed guidance and counseling about those problems and related limitations so they could become successfully employed. For applicants whose jobs were in jeopardy, counselors were often advised to make sure they showed a "lot of good counseling and guidance" and, therefore, were not simply purchasing a medical service, such as medical follow-up or a prosthesis.

Problematic cases occurred when a QC believed the applicant only needed a bill paid or that the counselor would not be providing counseling and guidance above and beyond what the doctor who was providing the medical services (such as treatment for high blood pressure) might provide. Uncertainty over substantial services was, in part, due to the agency's recent change in policy, as the following exchange in a case development staffing indicates:

Counselor 1: If ya'll agree that it's plan worthy. I have this client that is 20 years old. He's completed two years at [a technical school] in accounting, two-year degree. He was in an automobile accident, and he got a head injury which caused the loss of hearing in one ear. . . . He's got tinnitus which is that constant ringing all the time and it's driving him crazy. . . . Now he wants to go and get a four-year degree in accounting at [university], and he would like Voc Rehab's assistance. He meets economic need. Now, as far as substantial services, he needs, he *really* does need help in adjusting to that ringing in his ear, and also it's hard to go from bilateral hearing to unilateral hearing. And, you know, he's got a disability in my opinion, but I don't know if training is really the correct answer to his disability, and I just want ya'll's opinion.

QC: What do ya'll think?

Counselor 2: Yeah.

Counselor 3: Um hum.

Counselor 4: Wants to get a four-year degree in accounting?

Counselor 1: And he's already paid for two.

Counselor 3: That's what I think's a good case . . .

Counselor 2: I think it's a good case.

Counselor 4: Yeah, yeah, he's already paid for two of the years.

QC: Well, again now, now I see where [Counselor 1] is coming from. What about, what involvement are we going to have with this client? Is he going to need *our* involvement? And you need him for two years? He's already completed two. Are we going to be able to show our substantial involvement over a period of two years *other* than paying for tuition?

Counselor 2: Of course. Well, he's got the hearing loss so he's going to have to adjust to. She's going to be involved in that. She's going to be involved in getting him to study because once you lose something like that, to go back to school or anything else you try to do, you've got problems.

Counselor 1: And that's true. he might need some concrete counseling in areas of, you know, how to, where to sit in the class room, how to present that loss to his instructors so that they wouldn't turn their back on him when they're talking. It would be important for him to be able to look them straight in the face if at all possible. I'm scratching, I admit it, but . . .

QC: Don't, I mean, I think I got the feeling that you were not quite sure, you were . . .

Counselor 1: I'm not comfortable with my definition of substantial services probably. But I think It's an okay case, but I just wanted to check.

QC: Well, let's face it, a year ago it would have been written. You'd come in here and that would have been an afterthought to even staff it. Is that correct?

Counselor 1: Yeah, probably.

QC: Okay, now I think, this is to me, just the same as any other case that would be staffed in that if you, and of course, just like we went over in the case manual study that decision, that final decision, is yours. It's your opinion as to whether or not you are going to provide substantial services and you're able to show it.

Counselor 1: I think I can do that, I just . . .

QC: No problem then.

Counselor 1: I mostly kinda wanted to hear how ya'll felt and see what you said.

QC: I don't see any problem, you know. But, you know, just so we can get that documented as to substantial services that you're providing over that period of time. Sounds like a good case.

In order to establish what they were going to do, counselors *used* the rehabilitation staff and other professionals in the community. The professionals were a resource (though sometimes an obstacle) to be drawn upon in developing services. While counselors, not knowing what to do, often asked for and accepted the professionals' recommendations, they also requested or rejected recommended services, sometimes doing so even when they had initially approached the professionals with no preconceived plan of action. For example, in the case of an applicant whose abuse of alcohol was causing pancreatitis:

> The medical consultant noted that the counselor would need to counsel and guide well the applicant about that matter, perhaps even arranging for the applicant to be involved in Alcoholics Anonymous or some other program. Upon hearing that, the counselor asked the medical consultant to put in her recommendations something about the necessity for strong intervention in order for the applicant to stop drinking.

Also, after learning in a case development staffing group that if a counselor could tie the applicant's dental problems to his other disabilities, then the counselor might be able to provide treatment for the dental problem, the counselor went to the medical consultant (MC) seeking that "tie-in":

> *Counselor:* This is a multiple disability case. He's got about eight diagnoses under the basic medical. He's . . . diabetic, severe. He's got an umbilical hernia, obesity, . . . bad vision, and real severe dental problems. And, as you know it's kinda difficult for us to sponsor this kind of treatment. But I just staffed it in CDS, and they said if we can tie this in with these other disabilities, we stand a chance of being able to justify it and getting it done. He is in a lot of discomfort, a lot of pain with his teeth—inflamed gums.
>
> *MC:* And he is diabetic?
>
> *Counselor:* Uh huh. He takes insulin by needle. And I do have him a job . . . If I just, you know, get relief for him. . . . He's got pretty severe asthma. I got him on the desensitization program on that. . . . I think . . . with doing all those other things and not doing that [the dental] . . . it may not. . .
>
> *MC:* Just turn around on you, huh?
>
> *Counselor:* Uh huh. And I've got an internist's report. . . . It's hard to read.
>
> *MC:* Not much of a copy. . . . Well, from the dentist's description of his mouth he really has quite bad, he can't chew and the possibility of infection [spreading] from his gums, infected gums, is real with his diabetic condition, so I think we got a legitimate reason to . . .
>
> *Counselor:* OK. If you maybe would make a comment, you know, [MC: OK] in that reference [long pause as medical consultant writes]. I just feel real good about this man's attitude and his motivation. He could very easily keep getting food stamps and such as that, but he would rather work.

> Matter of fact, I think, . . . his checks from the social services were higher
> than his paychecks right now, but he just has a lot of self-pride and he
> wants . . . to work.

> *MC:* Well, I've said he needs to have dental work to improve general health,
> dash, poor, infected gums, source of infection, in this diabetic. Also,
> better nutrition will be received from improved dentation.

Counselors might also reject the professionals' recommended services, either because the applicant's circumstances had changed or
because the counselors did not believe the recommended services were
feasible. In either case, the counselors needed to justify why the
recommendations would not be followed.

> After a young female applicant had been kicked out of her family's house
> by her father, the counselor told the psychological consultant that she
> could not go along with his earlier recommendations for adjustment
> services because the applicant needed a job in order to support herself and
> her two children. The psychological consultant did not object and told the
> counselor that she did not need to staff the case with him, but that she
> should document in the case folder why his recommendations would not
> be followed.

Or, as one counselor noted of recommendations that she felt were "off
the wall" because nobody would have the time to manage the
recommended services:

> Most of the time you can justify it is not practical in terms of time or the
> client is desperately wanting to go to work and it's felt that work and a
> regular paycheck would be beneficial to the client's mental status. You
> also staff it with your peers, in CDS, and maybe come up with something
> that's a little bit more manageable and a little more practical. You can
> overrule what they say.

WORKING (WITH) THE APPLICANT

While the applicant's behavior and concerns (as well as sometimes
those of concerned third parties, such as family members) were
important throughout the making of a case, in the development of
services they were perhaps most crucial. In working (with) the applicants, counselors asked them, "What are we going to do?" and then
decided on a plan. Applicants "arrived" at the agency with widely
varying and more or less developed notions of what they wanted from

the agency. Some came with specific services in mind (such as eyeglasses or sponsorship in training at a postsecondary institution); whereas others had nothing in mind, perhaps coming in with no knowledge that they "needed" any service and certainly not knowing what the agency could provide. Because counselors took into account the desires of applicants (though they did not simply give in to those desires), those with an interest could be advocates for that interest.[13] Those who were not knowledgeable or who had no specific services in mind were more dependent upon the counselors' orientations to planning services (and doing their jobs).[14] Those orientations varied greatly.

Some counselors were "giveaway artists." They "automatically got everybody an eye exam, . . . automatically got everybody teeth, . . . automatically sent everyday to school," according to one counselor who took over some of these colleagues' caseloads, or "messes," as the counselor called them. In taking over such caseloads, the counselor was confronted with prior promises the counselor felt were inappropriate, if not illegitimate. The counselor noted of such a caseload:

> I had a lot of explaining to do to clients when I couldn't buy them glasses. "Well, [the counselor] said I was going to get glasses." Because in the [counselor's] mind, helping these people was getting them glasses. Unfortunately, legally we just can't buy glasses for all those people.

Colleagues who were critical of such an approach speculated as to why some counselors were "giveaway artists." Perhaps they were "meeting their own emotional needs." Or, "just coming out of the master's program in rehabilitation," they had a "very idealistic and long list of what rehabilitation could do" but were less concerned about organizational concerns, such as "meeting deadlines." The same idealistic and inexperienced counselors may have looked at what they did "more as social work than rehabilitation" (Euler, 1979). Or, as one counselor, who as a "brand new rookie" would "get you (the applicant/ client) anything you wanted [because] that was my job—to help you," explained:

> There are a lot of counselors who are not comfortable with themselves enough to look at a client and say, "I'm going to help you find a job by nagging you." Okay, they're going to say, "Well, why would this person come in here if all I'm gonna do is tell them to work? Why would they bother to come see me? But they'll keep appointments if I buy them work shoes or give them placement maintenance or something like that."

Such counselors gave and did not expect much in return.[15]

I did not see any counselors acting as "giveaway artists," though I observed some who were more willing to give and buy than others. Perhaps I did not observe any because either they had changed, as the counselor quoted above had, or they had left the agency. As one critic of giveaway artists remarked, "I don't know quite what the mind set of people like that is, but counselors like that, a lot of them aren't around anymore, too." Of course the agency itself was changing from bill paying (giveaway) to offering substantial services.

The critics of the giveaway artists took a no-nonsense, yet caring, approach to working with applicants (and clients), a "tough-love" approach.[16] They worked *within* an organization to *serve* people. Within those organizational concerns people could be helped. As one critic remarked,

> I'm trying to follow the policy of the agency the best I know it. . . . They want us to work towards placement, and that is . . . reflected in that they want us to work towards a certain number of placements. . . . And then within that framework I find that I have enough flexibility to help people that really need help.

In "following the agency's policy" to help people, these tough-love counselors typically did not make promises, did not push services on the applicants (and clients), but did expect the applicants to have a stake (often monetary) in their rehabilitation. Hence, applicants (and clients) would be "allowed" to pick up (some of) the medication tab, pay for books if the agency was paying for tuition, or cover the hospitalization costs if the doctor's fees were taken care of. One counselor explained:

> I would say, "Okay, I'll pay your tuition. Can you cover your books?" And nine times out of ten, a real motivated client is going to be tickled pink to get their tuition and they'll say, "Yeah, I could do that!" You know, and that's the way I'll do it. If you're fairly straightforward with them, "Okay, now look, I'm not going to pay for everything. You ought to have a little stake in this, too, don't you think? You're getting the education out of this." If they come in and expect me to foot the entire bill, like "Well, you're going to pay my gas, too, aren't you?" And I'll go, "Yeah, I didn't take you to raise" [a joke that the counselor was not the applicant's parent].

If the applicant did not ask for a service that was not essential to the rehabilitation process, the tough-love counselors did not offer it. One tough-love counselor remarked:

I don't offer a whole lot. In other words, if my clients want something, they're going to have to come out and ask for it, in terms of buying them things, you know, If they don't ask, I don't buy it.

By being straightforward, counselors minimized difficulties, though they certainly did not avoid all of them. Another tough-love counselor explained:

I have found that if I am straightforward with clients from the first moment I see them, I don't have any problem.... When they first sit in the chair, I say, "What is it you would like us to do?" "Well, I got my teeth." I say "Well, I'm sorry, the odds are we're not going to be able to help you with your teeth.... What else do you need?" "Well, I need a job and I have high blood pressure." I say, "Okay, I think I can help you with that."

Tough-love counselors were sensitive to the concerns of applicants, but they were sensitive within a context of organizational concerns and their own professional orientations. Some more than others would legitimately provide desired tangibles (such as eyeglasses) in order to work with and serve the applicant in other ways (such as counseling and guidance or psychotherapy).[17] By providing the tangible, a case could be made, an individual who needed help served, a successful closure achieved:

A young man was referred by his mother because the son needed glasses and the mother could not afford them. Suspecting an emotional problem, the counselor arranged a psychological evaluation where a "severe adjustment reaction" was diagnosed. The counselor made a "deal": The agency would buy the young man glasses if he went to psychotherapy sessions and "really put some effort into it." Apparently the young man did, because the student's guidance counselor called the rehabilitation counselor to inform the latter of how well the young man was doing, a "hundred percent change."

Nevertheless, in being sensitive to the concerns of the applicants, the tough-love counselors expected, as did the one quoted above, a commitment from the applicants. If tangibles were to be provided, then the applicants were expected to follow through with the other services. If, taking into account the wishes of the applicants, counselors adjusted what they felt were the most appropriate courses of action, then the applicants were expected to return to the original courses of action if the adjusted ones did not work.

An applicant who abused alcohol was originally scheduled to go to a state facility for long-term treatment [28 days]. However, due to a "very important job interview," the applicant wanted to begin the long-term treatment, leave for the interview, and then resume the treatment after the interview. After several calls to staff at the facility, the counselor learned that such could not be arranged. Although the counselor had an "uncomfortable feeling," a plan was developed for treatment of the applicant's alcohol abuse through a local agency and for job placement, with the contingency that if the alcohol abuse continued, then the applicant would go to the state facility for long-term treatment. The alcohol abuse continued, and subsequently the client did go to the state facility.

In working with the applicants, the tough-love counselors developed services with the applicants' working in mind. Placement was the biggest problem to one of them. If the applicants wanted to work ("they were pushing you real hard"), then counselors would not load them down with services they had not requested (and also did not need to address their handicaps) and would not fully take advantage of and/or that would do them a "disservice" because they needed the money. One tough-love counselor noted that you "don't argue" with the foul-smelling, poorly educated applicant with no recent work history, who does not want to go to "no stupid classes," does not "want to learn how to be clean," but is "satisfied to go to work part-time" at a convenience store because "you want him to go to work." Therefore, instead of providing a "lot of services," one provides the minimally necessary services to enable the applicant to work. If the applicants would not commit themselves to even the minimally necessary services, then no case could be made.

If it was a toss-up between between training or going "directly" to work, counselors were pleased if the applicants chose the latter. As one tough-love counselor who rarely trained applicants noted:

> Everybody needs retraining. . . . I'd love to be retrained, but the point is I don't need to be retrained. I'm quite capable of working [and most applicants with whom the counselor worked were also quite capable of working].

Thus counselors worked with applicants in deciding what they were going to do, but how they worked with applicants depended on counselors' orientations and applicants' actions. Similar, though certainly not identical, contrasts in orientations exist among other human service professionals, such as "caseload-oriented" and "applicant-oriented" approaches among intake workers in public welfare agencies (Zimmerman, 1966: 285-292). Counselors and other human service professionals may modify their orientations as they continue to confront the "tensions between capabilities and objectives" (Lipsky, 1980: 142-156) among their concerns, the clients' concerns, and their agencies' concerns.

Vocational Objective:
What Will (Can) the Applicant Do?

The vocational objective was the fourth element of the case, though it was not always the last to be established. Counselors had to establish that with the intended services there was a "reasonable expectation" that the applicant would become (or remain) employed in an appropriate position. Establishing an appropriate objective was the primary task typically faced by counselors.

If there was a reasonable expectation that the applicant could benefit vocationally from services, then counselors needed to establish an appropriate (and an alternate) vocational objective, appropriate with respect to the applicants' capabilities and disabilities. Generally the vocational objective was a position in competitive employment. Homemaker, sheltered workshop employee, family worker, and other "special occupations" were possibilities, though homemaker was the only "special occupation" with particular significance. In the past several years, closures in "special occupations" decreased in the agency from approximately 14 percent of all closures to approximately 6 percent, and almost all of these (approximately 90 percent) were homemaker closures.

Homemaker was a potentially problematic vocational objective (and closure; Guthrie et al., 1981). While it was a "legitimate" objective, the case manual stated somewhat contradictorily that "employment for pay can be considered a higher, although not exclusive goal," and "family status and earnings are not conditions of closure for the homemaker, nor are other factors such as the expectation that the vocational rehabilitation of the homemaker free another family member to engage in competitive employment." The manual continues, "Criteria for closing cases of clients as rehabilitated . . . do not bar such closure where job at closure may be homemaking even though the vocational objective and rehabilitation services were directed to other work," and "nothing in this policy should be interpreted as in any way encouraging the closing of a case as a homemaker in lieu of an unsuccessful closure due to the inability to obtain a competitive, vocational objective."

Homemaker was a potentially problematic objective because of the agency's mandated emphasis on work and the possibility that the label of homemaker was being used simply to "salvage" a case. Either the (female) applicant did not want to go to work, so homemaker would be the objective, or during the delivery of services new circumstances developed (such as pregnancy and birth) such that the client was not going to work, so the objective would be changed to homemaker. One counselor was advised that it would look better if the vocational objective were changed during the course of services from homemaker to a competitive job rather than vice versa. Hence homemaker should be listed as the first objective and the competitive job as the alternate. Further, there was continuing concern as to what substantial services would be and what services were actually provided to clients with homemaker as an objective. A new "homemaker program" provided by the agency only partially solved the problem.

The typical vocational objective was a position in competitive employment. Counselors were required to establish that the objective was appropriate to the applicant's capabilities and disabilities. What constituted satisfactory evidence for establishing the objective had changed over the years. While in the past a statement that the vocational objective was based on the "applicant's interest of long standing" or on a "vocational assessment counseling session" (a talk between the counselor and applicant) would have been acceptable, it was no longer. Instead, other evidence was usually used.

Counselors routinely used the expressed interest and the work history of adult applicants in establishing a vocational objective. For those who were unemployed at the time but wanted to return to a job they had done in the past or a similar one, the vocational objective became that job. For those who were employed but whose jobs were in jeopardy, maintaining the existing jobs became the vocational objective. However, when applicants had no significant recent work history—for example, students—or could not return to their previous jobs due to their disabilities, more investigation was needed to establish a vocational objective. Counselors arranged for an evaluation at the rehabilitation center or by an evaluator at their school program. I did not examine these evaluations (see Murphy and Ursprung, 1983), yet it was clear that counselors were not bound by them. They used the information provided in the evaluations, and even rejected the recommendations, in establishing the objectives for which they were ultimately responsible. For example:

> In developing a plan, the counselor was faced with the decision of which of three recommendations from the rehabilitation center would be used in establishing the primary and secondary vocational objectives. The evaluation report listed assembly line worker, electronics worker, and sewing machine operator. The counselor decided to list the assembly line worker as the first objective and the sewing machine operator as the second. She eliminated electronics worker after learning from the *Dictionary of Occupational Titles* the demands of the job in light of the applicant's high school education. Further, her applicant did not have a car and the bus routes did not include the electronics plants.

Or, if a counselor believed there was little hiring being done in the recommended field (such as "child care attendant, . . . work in a nursery school, that's just a real common vocational objective that all evaluators love, [but] nobody is hiring child care attendants"), then the counselor would reject the recommendations (though perhaps share them and the concerns with the applicant). Instead, the counselor might "know of something" that the applicant could do or, through the *Dictionary of Occupational Titles,* could find some similar jobs that require the same skills. Counselors reworked recommendations in order to use them.[18]

In establishing a vocational objective, counselors needed to avoid raising the concern that the objective was incompatible with the applicant's capabilities and limitations. As a QC explained:

> One of the first things we look at would be: Does the vocational objective itself—is it in line with the person's abilities? For instance, a case was staffed yesterday for an IWRP. It has not been written yet, in which the person is retarded, severely retarded. Well, not severely. I would say moderately retarded and with seizures. And vocational objective is going to be a carpenter's helper. Well, the first thing you think about is this waves a flag. Is the person going to be working around power saws . . .? Is he going to be climbing on ladders? Is he lifting trusses up in case they're doing some renovations and what have you? And this is where the counselor has to indicate that, yes, it's going to be as a carpenter's helper. However, this will be specialized placement in which the employer either knows the person or will know of the person's problem and the person will be working only on ground level, will not be working around any power machinery, and the counselor also indicates that the person is well

regulated for his seizures and takes his medication. He's only had maybe
two seizures in the past six months, and both times it was because of not
taking medication on a regular, routine basis. So these are the little things
you have to look for. I've had cases in the past where the counselor
accepted a yound lady with a hearing problem. Now, I think, as you
know, probably most all of us have a slight hearing problem to some
degree. It's not going to be perfect much the same as our vision is not
always perfect, but we compensate for it. If we are able to accept a person
with a hearing problem it must be such that the hearing is severe enough
that it will—that it is a vocational impairment. And, he accepted the
person based on that. Everything was going fine up to the point of
vocational objective. She was going to be—her objective was going to be a
music major in the piano or what have you. And this just doesn't ring a
bell. You—the feeling is that you have to have fairly good hearing in order
to—I mean this is hearing, this isn't seeing, and I know you can write
music, but you've still got to hear it. Of course, it was awfully hard to get
him to understand why this was not a legitimate vocational objective. It
would be the same as if you have a person with a back problem and it's,
let's just say that, it's severe enough that we are able to accept him, that he
has enough limitations—and then we turn right around and put him back
on the same type of work, whether it be a pulp-wood worker or someone
who has to do a lot of lifting and so forth. So, we're really not helping him
at all. All we're doing at that point would be to get him over this crisis, so
that he can go back and return to the same type of work and end up with
the next crisis.

Counselors handled the concerns about an inappropriate vocational
objective in several ways. The counselors might reassess the evaluation
in order to establish a more appropriate objective. Instead of secretary,
perhaps office helper would become the objective for an applicant with
an IQ score below 70. The primary and secondary objectives might be
reordered. Thus the vocational objectives of mail clerk and file clerk
were reordered for a client with a herniated disc, the reasoning of fellow
counselors being that the position of mail clerk might entail too much
bending and lifting. Selective placement, such as light-truck driver for
someone with back problems who could not lift heavy objects, might be
emphasized. An applicant might be retested with the hope that the new
score (on an IQ test perhaps) would be high enough to justify a
particular objective (and the training needed for that objective). Or, as in
the following example, several strategies might be employed:

The plan for an individual with "prior emotional problems" and who was
a "bit violent" (he had pulled a pharmacist across the pharmacy counter

when denied Valium) was returned by the state QC because the QC did not feel that he could function as a security guard, which was the first vocational objective and which had been based on prior experience. The counselor documented again that the case was staffed with the appropriate professional staff at a local mental health center who felt that with continued medication the applicant could function as a security guard. Further, the placement would be selective. "It was understood" that if the individual became a security guard, he would not be given a gun. He would only "monitor the premises." According to the counselor, this was the only way the objective of security guard could be retained.

Finally, vocational objectives in general, and not just homemaker in particular, were problematic. As I examine in the next chapter, clients did not always become successfully employed in one of the vocations chosen originally as an objective. When that occurred, counselors had to justify why there was a change in order to close the case successfully. Counselors used the objectives, particularly the secondary objective, as a hedge against the necessity of later amending the vocational objective. One counselor teased another for listing "accountant" and then "accounting clerk" as the primary and secondary objectives. For an applicant who had training in motel/hotel management and had taken a course in maintenance, the primary objective was to be a motel clerk. However, if the applicant could not "get a job as the apartment manager," then he would "try to get a job working as a maintenance man at an apartment" according to the counselor. Or, a counselor decided to list "sales representative" as the secondary objective for an applicant with an advanced degree in nutrition who was currently selling door to door, just in case a potential job as nutritionist, which would be the first objective, did not work out. Others felt that general, rather than specific, objectives (such as laborer, which to one counselor meant a "number of different occupations in which you would work with your hands" in contrast to "something like a sanitation worker") were more appropriate; clients, especially students, changed their interests, and the "specific" jobs were not always readily available. While the agency had moved toward specific objectives in the past several years, such a move was problematic to the counselors. Consequently, counselors recognized or were advised to be ready for the possibility that an amendment concerning the objective was likely to be needed later. Some wondered if there was perhaps too much made of establishing a vocational objective. For many clients who had few skills, an entry-level job of any kind would be "doing good." For others with skills, the job market was too tight for them to be so choosy.[19] Thus one counselor told his clients that the vocational objectives were not "binding because the job market [was] not that way" (that is, accommodating). Nevertheless, with the establishment of the vocational objective and the previous three elements of the case, a plan could be written.

THE PLAN

To make a case for their applicants successfully, counselors had to develop individualized written rehabilitation programs, IWRPs. These plans were the culmination of the counselors' investigative work. The one-page form contained an evaluation summary, which was covered by a flap and usually not seen by the applicant, in which the counselor described how the applicant's disability was vocationally handicapping and justified the vocational objective to be pursued. Beneath the summary, the counselor outlined intermediate goals, the criteria by which the goals would be determined to have been met, and the services to be provided in order to meet those goals. Counselors estimated the time of service to meet each of those goals, and identified the parties who were financially responsible for the services, such as the agency, the applicant, and/or a third party. The final goal was always successful performance for a minimum of sixty days (six months if self-employed) in the vocational objective. The intermediate goals and services were designed to address functional limitations, ways in which, as stated in the evaluation summary, the disability was vocationally handicapping. The plan and the supporting information in the case folder had to document the interrelationship of the four elements of the case—the disability, vocational handicap, services, and vocational objective. In doing so, two parts of the plan—the evaluation summary and the rehabilitation program—needed to be interrelated, too. As one QC explained:

> You gather all your information that's inside the folder. This is your information. And from that, you write the summary part of the IWRP. This shows all of those things, those problems which are handicapping to the person. Showing not only . . . symptoms of this, but you also have to indicate the maladaptive behavior or the problems to employment. You know, a person could have an emotional problem which causes him to cry, causes him to laugh inappropriately. OK, those are symptoms, but you have to indicate how that crying or laughing inappropriately affects

work. OK, once they do that up there, then down at the bottom of the IWRP, your goal, criteria, and service, you've got to show where you are either going to remove, reduce, or work around each of these functional problems. You take care of each of these functional problems. It's almost like a novel to the degree that you're starting out with removing this problem, removing this problem, improving the person here, right on down to the final chapter of the book which says "successful employment." So everything builds up to this final climax of successful employment.

Near the beginning of my research the agency developed the one-page form currently in use for the plan. In comparison to the previous plan, which was several pages long and duplicated materials in the case folder, the current form requires much less time for the counselor (and the casework assistant) to fill out. Some counselors and supervisory staff noted that if you knew what you wanted to do, it could take as little as five minutes to write the plan.

However, the change to the new format did lead to some uncertainty regarding how the plan should be written. Training sessions were held to educate the counselors. "Trial and error" (that is, writing plans and having them returned by the state office) was instructive, too. Some counselors, particularly new ones, at times used past, successful plans as models in writing present ones.

In writing plans, counselors needed to be (sufficiently) specific about how the disability vocationally handicapped the applicant and how those limitations were to be addressed through the substantial services of the agency. There was no hard-and-fast rule as to when that specificity had been achieved. If someone had a back condition, then to note that the individual "cannot lift over 25 pounds" was much more specific than to say the person "has a lot of pain," the latter being both vague and a description of a symptom, rather than a limitation. However, statements that were too specific might create problematic commitments for the counselors. One counselor noted without pinning herself down:

> I'm possibly broad with what I say in my plans because if you aren't, then sometimes you can pin yourself down really bad. [What do you mean?] Need to leave yourself flexibility. I don't know if I can give you specifics. Something I learned in . . . years with the agency.

Specifics of not pinning yourself down might include "weight loss" as an intermediate goal without stating a specific amount of weight to be lost or "tools, if needed," as a service to be provided.

Counselors, like other human service professionals (Gubrium, 1980a), routinized the writing of plans. The agency's guidelines regarding how plans were to be written (such as the specific order of goal, criteria, and service) helped to routinize this activity. One counselor noted that

> IWRP does not leave much room for literary personality, "as determined by, through," you know, all this stuff. So you pretty well have to put it down. Whereas before, when you had the . . . [previous format], you could pretty well word it.

In routinizing the writing of plans, counselors used standardized phrasing. "Based on client's experience," "negatively affects work performance," and "based on case folder documentation" were frequently used phrases. One counselor even noted that as long as he used the "same words" in writing plans, he experienced no difficulty. The standardized wording often came from previous plans that had been approved. Other counselors routinely included a specific goal (or goals) on their plans, such as "improve interview skills." One QC told a group of counselors that he was shown several plans by officials at the state office that read almost identically, and that this was inappropriate. At least one counselor modified the wording of plans slightly so that they would not read so similarly, a practice of other human service professionals as well (Gubrium and Buckholdt, 1982: 146). However, the counselors claimed that the agency's practice of returning plans in which they had shown some "creativity" (that is, in which they had not followed the standard pattern) put them in a bind: Standardize and have plans that read similarly or individualize (too much) and the plans might be returned.

I suspect that much of this dilemma concerned the distinction between style and substance. The agency wanted the style of the plans to be similar but the substance to be individualized. However, many counselors, especially those who managed speciality caseloads, routinely worked with individuals with similar problems (such as alcohol problems, hearing impairments, mental retardation, and mental health problems). Consequently, the substance of what they said was similar from case to case. Counselors and casework assistants spoke often at case development staffings of "another one of my [or another one of his or her] _____ plans," where the blank might be filled in with: "C and G" (counseling and guidance), job placement, and follow-up; purchase of a hearing aid, "C and G," and follow-up; or treatment at the (hospital), "C and G," tools if needed, job placement, and follow-up. As one counselor said of cases involving applicants who were mentally retarded,

> [The cases] are pretty standard . . . generally adjustment and placement. You know, they are usually healthy. You usually give [a] vocational evaluation on them and get a baseline of what kind of skills they've got. Either put them in my program here or in the workshop to build up their work skills, their work tolerance, their appearance, interview skills. And then when they've pretty well demonstrated they're ready to go to work, then we place them. Don't generally step out of that line hardly at all unless there's maybe a medical problem.

Of course, the C and G, adjustment, and placement in a vocational objective *might* vary considerably, but on paper the plans were similar.

While there may have been little "literary license" available to counselors in writing plans, they recognized that plans could be written and rewritten to make as strong a case as possible for the applicants' eligibility. Some counselors joked at one case development staffing about writing plans that were accurate *and* would be approved by the state QC. To make as strong a case as possible, counselors were advised to, or did, pay attention to the four elements of a case, particularly substantial services. For example, counselors were advised to split "job location" from "job follow-up" as two separate goals and to state clearly the ways in which placement would be pursued (such as a computer search involving listings with Job Service, newspaper advertisements, and employer contacts). Counselors might be advised to word or reword their plans so that substantial services were indicated clearly. For example:

> An applicant with a "hip problem" had been evaluated and, according to the counselor, finally realized that everything was "alright" with him except the hip. The applicant had worked as a mechanic and service station worker but would like to do "brake jobs" and a "little starter repair and that kind of thing" in his small shop. The plan was to provide several visits to an orthopedist for the hip, guidance and counseling, and placement. The supervisory professional who was "leading" the staffing questioned the counselor as to whether the work the applicant was returning to was "lighter" than the previous work. Assured that it was, the supervisory professional rcommended that the counselor emphasize that fact in the "write-up."

One counselor claimed routinely to state as a goal for clients "to do well on interviews" because this was achieved through the counselor's guidance and counseling, which became part of the substantial services being provided. In discussion of a case concerning an applicant with psoriasis, another counselor suggested that if the counselor handling the case were to indicate as the first intermediate goal "to improve the applicant's self-concept," then the plan would "go through" because many people assume that those with psoriasis have poor self-concepts. And after the state QC returned a plan in which "low back pain" had been mentioned, the counselor who had written the plan substituted the phrase "lumbar strain," which was in a medical report. The counselors' strategies in all of these were not to "make up," but to "make strong" the cases for applicants to those who would review the cases (see Gubrium, 1980a: 664-666).

In counselors' making as strong a case as possible, applicants were to be involved in the development of the IWRP. As one QC noted, in the past counselors might have been "secretive" about the plans, telling clients what was to be done as each step was approached. However, the Rehabilitation Act of 1973 required that applicants were to be involved in the development of their plans (Bitter, 1979).[20] Their involvement could vary greatly from the mentally retarded school applicants, whose active contributions were relatively modest, to the adults who knew what they wanted to do and how the agency might be able to help them (for example, through training). As noted earlier, counselors did take into account the concerns of applicants, and, therefore, applicants who were knowledgeable and/or assertive were more involved in the development of their plans than those who were less competent advocates.

In the actual writing of the plan, the ideal, according to one QC, would be for the counselor to have the applicant come into the office and write the IWRP in the applicant's presence. Some counselors did so, though one who did felt that most applicants "couldn't care less about that IWRP."[21] Others prepared the plan beforehand and then arranged for the applicant to come into the office to sign it after the two reviewed it. One counselor claimed that it made little sense to "trick" applicants into signing plans involving services with which they did not agree because they would not follow through and the counselors would not get credit for successful closures. And in retrospect one counselor realized that having uninterested applicants sign IWRPs did not work to the counselor's "advantage in the long run." They, too, did not follow through.

Finally, while counselors wrote plans with the hope that the clients would become successfully employed, counselors knew that such hopes were not always realized. At times, counselors wrote plans knowing that it was uncertain whether the closure would be a "26" or a "28," a success or a failure.[22] Some were not certain whether the applicant would become employed, but they would try. For some caseloads, such as the specialty caseload involving public offenders (see Chapter 6), that uncertainty was typical. The counselor in charge expected many closures to be "28s" and (unfortunately) was not disappointed. The number of failures often rivaled the number of successes. And, as one counselor explained, counselors were faced with goals for the number of plans written during the fiscal year as well as for the number of successful closures. No doubt some plans were written with the former goal in mind and only a hope for the latter.

COOLING OUT THE WOULD-BE CLIENT[23]

While counselors opened cases with the hope of making them, they were not always successful. Some applicants were determined not to be eligible for services, and others did not cooperate sufficiently for eligibility to be determined. When counselors opened cases but later closed them because the applicants were determined not to be eligible for services, counselors faced a potentially problematic situation: Applicants had sought help but were to be denied it. Counselors attempted to cool out the ineligible applicants, to mollify their disappointment with them and/or their agency. Counselors did so both in anticipation of the problem as well as when the situation actually arose.

Counselors anticipated the potential problem of applicants' not being eligible for services. Therefore, they often explained to the applicants that they could not "promise anything" until the applicants were evaluated thoroughly. Some shared their doubts with the applicants regarding their eligibility but arranged a medical evaluation anyway. However, from the complaints of counselors who were assigned cases previously handled by others, and from the advice of one QC to some counselors, it was clear some counselors had made promises or implied promises that had caused or could cause difficulty. The QC advised:

We should not basically promise people things until we fully evaluate . . .
We have at times made them feel that they were eligible, and we were, even
though [we were] not coming out and say[ing], "I promise you such and
such," we've said it in such a way that they take this as a promise.

Counselors might "sell" referrals on the benefits of being involved with
the agency, but they needed to do so without making promises that
might later be impossible to keep. Apparently some counselors at times
failed in that task.

If, after evaluating the applicants, counselors decided the applicants
were not eligible, then they tried to deflect the applicants' actual or
potential disappointment from them and/or the agency. They did so by
denying personal responsibility for the unwanted decision and/or by
providing alternatives to the agency's services, which were now unavail-
able. In denying personal responsibility for the unwanted decision,
counselors attempted to explain to the applicants the rules and
regulations of the agency, the evaluation procedures undertaken, and
the results that led to the applicants' not being eligible. Applicants were
told it was not the counselors' fault the applicants were not eligible, that
they were "bound by the rules of . . . [the] agency," or the evaluations
made by *other* professionals found not enough seriously wrong with the
applicants. The applicants should be pleased that *their* disabilities were
not severe. Counselors might even provide additional evaluations as a
way of demonstrating to the applicants that they were indeed trying to
help the applicants be served by the agency. As one counselor explained
about an applicant who had complained of "problems with his ears,"
and nothing "significant" had been found through evaluation:

He wasn't satisfied at all until he saw Dr. [name] that second time, but I
think he feels like he had a thorough evaluation now, although he wasn't
too pleased.

Counselors often tried to provide alternatives to applicants who were
to be denied the agency's services. One counselor remarked, "I never try
to cut off and leave a client standing without some direction."
Alternatives might include informal counseling, help in completing a
job application, referrals to other community agencies, or discussion of
how to apply for disability benefits from the Social Security Administration (perhaps accompanied by a supportive letter) if the applicant
was "too severe" for the vocational rehabilitation agency. For example,
one counselor explained:

I worked with a client last year that wanted to go to school and turned out not to be eligible. His handicap was just not severe enough for our agency to really work with.... He didn't really have a substantial handicap. So, in this particular instance he had no idea of how he could go to school. I informed him about the . . . grants there at school, and he went and applied for those grants, was eligible and accepted, and is . . . now at [a technical college].... [He is] doing super, making A's, working hard, [and is] very excited.

When cooling out ineligible applicants, counselors did not simply deny responsibility for refusing services, but often provided alternatives to the applicants that served the applicants well.

MAKING A CASE AGAINST THE APPLICANT

Detectives often find it difficult, if not impossible, to make a case if those seeking help do not cooperate. When victims (and witnesses) do not cooperate, law enforcement detectives may drop cases or not even undertake them. Rehabilitation counselors faced a similar concern in working their cases.

Many cases led nowhere. Applicants did not follow through with the necessary evaluations and appointments so counselors could make cases in their behalf. Counselors faced a dilemma. The agency realized it could not force applicants "to take its services," but it expected counselors to show sufficient effort to provide services. However, because counselors handled a large number of cases, they did not want to waste their efforts on those who were not following through. As one counselor remarked, "When you have so many clients to work with, you don't just keep pounding and pounding and pounding."

While counselors could not "make a case" for an applicant against the applicant's will, it was not always clear what that will was. Missed appointments and failure to keep in contact might be a sign of a lack of interest, but not necessarily. Unresponsiveness and irresponsibility were often important aspects of an applicant's disability and, specifically, of a vocational handicap. Therefore, counselors could not and did not simply close an applicant's case if the applicant missed a single appointment or failed to respond to a counselor's letter. Instead, counselors were required to establish a case against the applicant, to demonstrate that "reasonable" attempts had been made to obtain the applicant's participation in the rehabilitation process, but that due to the applicant's behavior such had not been possible. The case would be "08-ed."

While there was no formal rule as to when counselors closed unresponsive applicants' cases, counselors relied on several rules of thumb and other strategies to "08" such cases. If applicants missed several appointments (for example, for a medical examination) without providing adequate reasons, counselors would be likely to close those cases. Though it was certainly not as simple as "three strikes (missed appointments) and you're out," counselors seemed to use three missed appointments as a rough guideline in making their decisions. One counselor did not close an applicant's case until the applicant had missed *six* appointments with the staff psychologist. This elicited an exclamation from a colleague regarding the patience of the counselor, a clear indication that offering six chances was out of the ordinary.

However, it was not just several missed appointments, but the fact that applicants lacked adequate reasons for those misses that was important. For example:

> In one case development staffing, a counselor staffed a case for a colleague who was not present. The colleague intended to close the case of an applicant who had missed two appointments for psychological testing and one for a medical examination. However, because there was no indication in the colleague's field notes as to why the applicant had missed the appointments, and because the applicant had "problems galore" [she was 18 years old with four children, and had an eye removed], the staffing team decided to ask the counselor to find out what was "going on" with the applicant.

Or, as one counselor explained about applicants who missed appointments:

> If they call before and they say, "The car is broken down. I'm not going to be able to keep it," that's one thing. But if they miss it, and they don't call, and you have to track them down, that is something else again.

Counselors also interpreted applicants' actions as indicating inadequate reasons for missed appointments. Reasons for *continued* missed appointments might retrospectively be interpreted by counselors as excuses and the case would be closed. Applicants who swore they would keep a rescheduled appointment but did not might have their cases closed. In a similar manner Work Incentive Program counselors use clients' promises of future cooperation to undermine "future appeal [s] to extenuating circumstances" (Miller, 1983: 147). When rehabilitation counselors warned applicants that they needed to keep rescheduled appointments and if they did not their cases would be closed, their cases were often closed when they failed to keep the appointments. If after several missed appointments the counselors were unable to contact the applicants, the counselors made a "home visit" and left their cards, even though they did not see the applicants; then the applicants' failure to get in touch with the counselors would become grounds for closing their cases. Applicants' actions often spoke more clearly than their words.

Just as applicants needed to provide "reasonable" justification for missing appointments so counselors would not close their cases, counselors needed to justify closing applicants' cases. Instead of making a case for the applicants, they made a case against the applicants. Some cases were stronger than others. If counselors were able to contact their applicants personally and the applicants expressed no interest in further services, then the cases were closed. Such "direct refusal of services" was a stronger justification than a "home visit with a card left," which was stronger than several missed appointments. To build a stronger case for closing applicants' cases, counselors might set up "hoops," as one counselor called them, for applicants to jump through. If they failed to jump through the hoops, then the counselors would have justification for closing the cases. For example, an applicant failing to respond to a "contact card" (a postcard asking the recipient to contact the counselor) was not a particularly strong justification for closing the case. Instead, as one counselor suggested, an appointment could be set for the applicant to meet with the counselor. Failure to keep that appointment (failure to jump through the hoop) was a stronger justification for closing the case. Arranging an evaluation at the rehabilitation center or offering its services was used as a hoop by counselors to obtain a stronger justification for closing the case if the applicant failed to follow through or declined services. If the applicant did follow through, then the hoop served to get the case moving again. Thus counselors not only made cases for their applicants, but also against those who did not cooperate.[24]

CONCLUSION

Law enforcement detectives, rehabilitation counselors, and other human service professionals work cases in order to do their jobs—

solving crimes or serving citizens. After opening cases, rehabilitation counselors tried to make a case for applicants through the often routine development, organization, and use of information. If they were not successful, then counselors either "cooled out" disappointed applicants or made a case against uncooperative applicants. If counselors were successful, then applicants became clients, individuals who were eligible for the agency's services. Yet, cases that were successfully made might vary greatly. Some were "good" cases: The clients were motivated to cooperate and go to work, substantial services were clearly needed and could be provided, the cost might be low, and the "turnover" might be quick (the case would be closed successfully in several months). Other cases were "shaky." Due to the severity of the clients' disabilities or their lack of work experience or commitment, the counselors were uncertain about the outcome of the cases. They would be difficult cases, perhaps time-consuming and filled with setbacks.[25] Thus cases that were successfully made, whether "good" or not, were still far from being closed successfully; and some would not be. Therefore, once counselors made cases, they needed to conclude them.

NOTES

1. Law enforcement detectives screened out patrol reports of crimes, too. Detectives gave no or relatively little investigative attention to cases seen to be phony, "little," without leads, or not prosecutable (Sanders, 1977: 84-99). However, detectives might initiate some investigation before characterizing a case as one of these types. How detectives characterized cases, particularly in terms of being "little" or "big," depended on the typical cases the detectives received. For example, batteries were "little" cases for a major crimes detail, but they were important for a juvenile detail because that detail typically received such crimes as petty theft and malicious mischief.

2. In relatively fewer cases, counselors might screen out referrals after talking with the referral source or after observing the referral in an institutional setting without directly contacting the referral.

3. The major reason given by counselors for preferring to work or not to work with particular types of disabilities was the "speed and ease of success in achieving vocational rehabilitation" (Goldin, 1966). Consequently, perhaps counselors ranked persons with cancer as least likely to be served by them relative to persons with paraplegia, heart disease, and renal failure (Pinkerton and Nelson, 1978). Similarly, intake workers in a welfare department preferred simple cases over time-consuming, complicated cases (Prottas, 1979: 37-38).

4. Preadmission screening in a rehabilitation hospital could also be problematic because the charts and records ("paper referrals") sent to the hospital might be " 'in-

complete,' 'confusing,' or even 'misleading' " (Gubrium and Buckholdt, 1982: 129). Additional checking might be necessary.

5. During initial and subsequent interviews with (potential) clients, rehabilitation counselors focused primarily on gathering or giving information (Farley and Rubin, 1980).

6. A study of counselors in a southern state indicated that initial interviews ranged from 3 to 60 minutes, with an average of 24 minutes (Farley and Rubin, 1980).

7. Parole officers use the initial interview with their parolees in determining how much, if any, trouble they can expect from their parolees (McCleary, 1978: 109-110).

8. Experienced intake workers in public welfare agencies routinely use a stance of skepticism when confronting applicants. Workers come to believe that applicants may try to manipulate the agency (Zimmerman, 1966: 219-231).

9. One counselor advises colleagues not to test the motivation of referrals by giving them the application and seeing if they return it. That only "needlessly bogs down the process" (Willey, 1979: 156).

10. In a recent fiscal year, approximately two-thirds as many cases as were accepted for services were closed "08," (not accepted). In previous years as many, if not slightly more, cases were closed "08" as were accepted for services. In the same recent fiscal year mentioned above, approximately 9 percent of the "08s" were due to unfavorable medical prognosis or too severe handicaps, 20 percent to a lack of a disabling condition or vocational handicap (which, according to a state-level professional, would be more likely to occur on an inexperienced counselor's caseload), 10 percent to inability to locate/contact the applicant (or the applicant had moved), 55 percent to refusal of further services or failure to cooperate, and the remaining cases were closed due to the applicant's death, transfer to another agency, or institutionalization (for example, in prison).

11. In a two-state study, counselors and medical consultants disagreed about several procedures: making referrals for specialized examinations and treatments, involvement in making a preliminary diagnosis, determining the extent to which a client was following a doctor's orders, determining the extent of vocational handicap and eligibility, and deciding whether or not an applicant was too disabled to benefit from the agency's services. Each group wanted more control over these procedures than the other was willing to grant (Klein et al., 1982).

12. According to the case manual, a "substantial handicap to employment" existed when a

physical or mental disability (in light of attendant medical, psychological, vocational, educational, and other related factors) impedes an individual's occupational performance, by preventing his obtaining, retaining, or preparing for employment consistent with his capacities and abilities.

13. In response to case abstracts, rehabilitation counseling master's degree students and rehabilitation counselors in rehabilitation facilities and state agencies consistently, if also modestly, developed services based on their perceptions of clients' needs. However, as a group, state-agency counselors did not provide personal-social adjustment training or work adjustment training. Respondents with less work experience did (Crystal, 1981). Thus counselors' orientations vary individually and seemingly across work environments and according to experience.

14. Street-level bureaucrats can control the distribution of benefits to applicants through their control of information. This works most smoothly when applicants are not knowledgeable or aggressive. Those who are knowledgeable and aggressive can realize their demands as well as disrupt the street-level bureaucrats' work. Therefore, such applicants are often disliked (Prottas, 1979: 40-41, 115, 130-131, 137-141).

15. In human service agencies, clients may coopt the human service professionals. Rather than impersonally enforcing the rules of their agencies, the professionals "overidentify" with some of their clients. Consequently, they fail to enforce rules or break rules in order to benefit the clients (McCleary, 1978: 123-124).

16. The term "tough-love" was applied by one counselor to her approach to rehabilitation counseling. It was taken from the name of a "program for parents troubled by unacceptable 'teenage' behavior" (York et al., 1982: 13).

17. A critic of state vocational rehabilitation agencies argues that most clients do not want counseling (Olshansky, 1976). Similarly, a federal review of rehabilitation practices revealed that counselors believed that many of their clients would not be interested in participating in the agency's program if tangibles, such as paid medical bills, were not provided (GAO, 1978).

18. While the majority of rehabilitation counselors surveyed in the Southeast found vocational evaluations helpful, most of those who were "satisfied" found the evaluations only "somewhat helpful." Further, approximately two-fifths of the counselors felt, to varying degrees, that clients did not know any more about what jobs they could do when they finished the evaluations than when they started, and that evaluators typically recommended the same few jobs (McDaniel, 1979).

19. Perhaps consequently, a federal review several years ago of the state agency I observed found that documentation in the case folders frequently failed to indicate that vocational assessment was a significant area of deliberation between the counselor and applicant.

20. Due to the concern with applicants' involvement in developing their plans, a blank IWRP signed by the applicant was grounds for a counselor's immediate dismissal from the agency. I witnessed and was told about counselors who, when initially meeting the referral/applicant, had the individual sign a blank IWRP. During the few times I observed that happen, the counselor was not being secretive with the referral/applicant. Instead, the counselor discussed with the individual the latter's vocational interests and the kinds of services the agency could provide. Afterwards, the counselor justified such action by explaining that it was done to serve the individual better. Due to the nature of the referral, evaluative materials on which to build a case were available. However, it might be difficult for the counselor to find the individual's home in order to develop the IWRP and have it signed, or it might be difficult for the applicant to come to the counselor's office to take care of that matter in a timely manner. Further, particular services (which I will not mention due to concerns about counselor anonymity) could be arranged and provided to the client because a plan had been signed. Such an arrangement also served the counselor, saving the counselor from expending additional time and effort. In these few cases both the counselor and the applicant "seemed" to benefit.

21. A pilot study indicated that increased applicants' involvement in the development of the IWRP did not increase their satisfaction with agency services (Rubin, 1975: 179-180). If clients did not care, perhaps administrators did. Not surprisingly, rehabilitation counselors have viewed the IWRP as an organizational attempt to control their activities (Smits and Ledbetter, 1979).

22. Models have been developed to predict rehabilitation successes and failures. A recent model, using demographic, disability, work history, and public assistance

information correctly predicted the outcome for approximately 60 percent of the cases reviewed, a slightly lower percentage than that of cases closed successfully. Thus taking a chance on all the cases, as the counselors had done, led to a slightly better prediction than did the model (Worrall and Vandergroot, 1980, 1982).

23. Victims of a confidence game, the marks, who might complain to the police or otherwise create problems for the operators of the con, need to be managed. They are cooled out. The cooler attempts to "define the situation for the mark in a way that makes it easy for him to accept the inevitable and quietly go home" (Goffman, 1952: 452). Not only marks, but others who involuntarily lose a status or a claim to a status may need to be cooled out as well. For example, consolation may be needed by those who apply for the services of a human service agency but are denied those services or those who feel a wrong has been done to them because a crime has been committed but the police do not seem to care. In the latter cases detectives may "PR" (public relations) the cases by contacting the victims and pretending to look for suspects or explaining to the victims that little can be done (Sanders, 1977: 97-98).

24. During the course of my research, one strategy used by counselors, the "ten-day letter," became prohibited. This form letter typically stated that, in order for the agency to serve the recipient of the letter, the recipient needed to be involved in the vocational rehabilitation process. Therefore, if the recipient did not contact the counselor by a certain date (usually within ten days, though it could be two weeks, thirty days, or some other time period), then the recipient's case would be closed. Some counselors used the letter as a bluff to try to spur the applicant's interest, without actually closing the case if the applicant did not respond. Others personalized the letter. Instead of using a photocopied form letter, the counselors tailored a letter to the applicant's specific failure (such as failure to enter the workshop as scheduled), with the implication that failure to contact the counselor would mean the applicant was no longer interested in the agency's services. Personalizing such letters, however, took more time than using a form letter. Supervisory staff saw the "ten-day letter" as a "bit negative." It did not indicate sufficient effort on the part of the counselors to provide services, but instead was a threat to deny services. Failure to meet a scheduled appointment would be just as effective in determining the applicant's lack of interest as would failure to respond to a "ten-day letter," according to one supervisory staff member. Scheduling an appointment, however, was an offer of services, not a threat to deny them.

25. Other human service professionals as well as detectives develop conceptions of "good" cases, "ideal" patients, and the like (Sanders, 1980: 94-105; Gilsinan, 1982: 155-162; Gubrium and Buckholdt, 1982: 31-33, 36).

4

CONCLUDING CASES

Detectives have done their job when they have solved a case to their satification, identified a suspect, and, where appropriate and possible, have the suspect in custody. The case is cleared and likely to be closed. If a suspect is released on a "technicality," detectives "do not assume that the suspect was innocent and begin again to look for the culprit" (Sanders, 1977: 81). Rarely is new evidence introduced at a trial that leads detectives to question their assumption of the suspect's guilt. While failure of the suspect to be convicted may concern them, detectives rarely take it as an indication of their failure to do their job. "Detectives see themselves and not the courts as the most reliable judge of a suspect's innocence or guilt" (Sanders 1977: 81). For the most part, when law enforcement detectives have made a case, then they have done their job.[1] Not so for rehabilitation detectives.

Rehabilitation counselors have not finished their job when they have successfully made a case for their applicants. Making a case is only part of working cases, though much work has gone already into the cases. When cases have been made *and* successfully closed, rehabilitation counselors have then finished their job. Counselors work cases to serve clients; detectives do so to solve crimes. The difference here, between law enforcement and rehabilitation detectives is, of course, that the former primarily process people, while the latter process *and* change people. Like many other human service professionals, rehabilitation counselors not only process people (that is, establish their eligibility or ineligibility), but also serve them with the intent of changing them. Thus rehabilitation counselors not only attempt to "catch the criminals," but to "correct" them as well. They do both detective work and correctional work. Yet in doing correctional work, rehabilitation counselors continue their investigative activities. They continue to work the cases to ultimately conclude them.

In concluding cases, counselors provided their clients services enabling them to remain or become successfully employed. Counselors provided services in order to *place the clients*. After following the clients' progress to ensure their successful employment, counselors *closed the cases*. However, many cases did not proceed uneventfully to closure, and a significant number were not successfully closed. In either case, counselors *managed these problematic cases*. And the tale of each case, from opening to closure, was documented in the *record*.

While counselors provided a variety of services, sometimes a great many, to clients, I do not focus directly on those services. As I noted in the Introduction and in Chapter 1, while frameworks help us make sense of our observations and give meaning to what we include, they also necessitate that we exclude or give less attention to other matters. Further, many of the services provided to the clients were provided not by the counselors but by others inside and outside the agency. However, I do discuss the provision of services as I attempt to make sense of my observations concerning counselors' methods of concluding cases, but I do so within the metaphor of dective work.

PLACING CLIENTS

Placing clients was the "bottom line" in vocational rehabilitation counseling. As one counselor explained to me, though he did not want me to tape-record that portion of the interview, it did not matter how effective a counselor was in counseling clients, providing individual attention, or arranging for services, what counted to the agency and to (most of) the counselors was "getting clients back to work." In the past, when the agency was more heavily involved in "paying bills," placement was not as great a concern because many clients were then employed, their disability being a jeopardy to their employment. With the shift in policy, placement became a much greater concern to the agency and to the counselors. In contrast, the above-mentioned counselor described a former colleague:

> He just said, "I've done everthing else. I don't see that [job placement is] part of my job" [counselor laughs]. He was proud of that. He had been

with the agency about . . . three years. He's not with us anymore. He didn't leave for that reason, but, you know, he said, "I made my referrals. I referred them to Job Service. . . . . I take care of all their physical needs. Now they can handle it from here." But that's got to change.

Indeed it did appear to be changing. A state-level administrator explained that placement was going to be the "biggest, single" focus in the coming years. Baseline data concerning the degree of counselor involvement in placement was then being collected. After it was collected and assessed, the state-level administrator planned to establish guidelines for improving the degree of counselor involvement in placement.

The agency's conern with placement and the contrast between the counselor mentioned above and his former colleague, point to the ambivalent position of placement in the rehabilitation process and among rehabilitation counselors (Flannagan, 1974). While vocational rehabilitation has not been achieved until the client has been successfully placed, counselors do not particularly relish placement (Zadny and James, 1977a: 154). While they spend relatively little time on it (approximately between 4 percent and 7 percent) (Zadny and James, 1976), they feel it constitutes a substantial part of their job, though not as substantial as administrators feel it is or should be, and they report that they have "insufficient time to carry out placement activities with about one-third of their clients," especially those that involve direct contact with employers (which they also feel is of less importance to their job than other placement activities, such as placement counseling) (Emener and Rubin, 1980: 62). Counselors would "willingly have a special placement counselor perform" placement activities (Muthard and Salomone, 1969: 115). However, in comparison to counselors of a decade or two ago, present-day counselors are more likely to believe that job placement activities that involve working with clients have become a large part of their job (Emener and Rubin, 1980). While placement's ascribed significance has increased, the ambivalence surrounding it remains.[2] That ambivalence became evident at times in how counselors "did" placement.

Placement involved a wide variety of activities by the counselors and clients. Much of it included detective work regarding the *identification of job leads* and the *management* of clients in relation to those leads. Both concerns were handled in various ways.

Identifying Leads

Leads differ as to how effective, efficient, and available they are in enabling clients to secure employment. Some leads, such as want ads and other well-advertised openings, are readily available, but often not very promising (Zadny and James, 1978). Too many other people use them. Others, such as a special relationship with an employer, are less available but also more effective. The inside connection makes the difference. Counselors identified job leads in various ways.

With the emphasis noted in Chapter 2 on "marketing," the agency became more concerned with "selling" itself to employers. By making employer contacts, counselors hoped to develop not only a source of referrals for "troubled" employees, but contacts that later might be useful in placing clients. "Marketing" became implemented at the end of my research. Consequently, I cannot comment much on it. Suffice it to say that counselors who had worked for some time in the local area would have been likely to develop more employer contacts than less experienced counselors. Some counselors faced making employer contacts with apprehension because they did not know how they would be received. Would the meeting with the employer go well or not (Flannagan, 1974)? Without previous employer contacts, counselors might feel uncomfortable contacting an employer on their own regarding job leads. As one inexperienced counselor explained:

> I don't have a lot of the employer contact. If I stay with the agency a long time, I might develop those, but right now basically how I do it [job placement] now is I try to contact employers as my clients contact them. . . . I don't feel like I can pick up the phone and call someone. I'm sure . . . some of the counselors around here can do that.

"Marketing" could be seen, in part, as formalizing what some counselors had been doing on a more informal basis. Through past dealings with employers, membership in civic organizations, relations with other professionals in the agency who had developed their own contacts, direct contact with employers when no previous relationship had existed, friends of family members, and contacts made at social occasions, such as parties or "bar hopping," counselors developed employer contacts, one source of job leads. Thus, even when counselors were "off duty," they may have done their duty.

Counselors regularly used many strategies in addition to developing employer contacts to identify job leads. Newspaper want ads were scanned regularly by counselors and passed on to clients. The local Job Service Office, which attempted to find employment for the un-employed, could be helpful. Office colleagues who knew of possibilities might inform one another when none of their clients could use the tip. Thus friendships among colleagues in the office could prove important. However, with the agency's marketing strategy, job leads were being shared among counselors in their job development groups. Clients who knew of openings and the counselors' recent successes in placing clients in particular fields and companies also led to job leads. "Inside" contacts, such as a family member, a former client who was grateful for services rendered, or a manager who was personally known, were all used in identifying job possibilities. Government agencies or private companies sometimes contacted the rehabilitation agency and specifically requested an employee who was disabled, sometimes even specifying the disability. My suggestions were also used in identifying job leads, and in one case it turned out to be a successful lead. "Effective rehabilitation counselors . . . usually developed and cultivated informal networks of job informants" (Wright, 1980: 649).[3]

Managing the Client

Counselors needed not only to identify job leads, but also to manage their clients in relationship to those leads. In doing so, their aim was to meet their goals of successful closures, as well as to place individual clients. If handled inappropriately, the particular placement of any individual client (or the general placement of clients) might lead to an individual success, but to a general failure. Efforts expended inefficiently or unwisely might jeopardize both the placement of other clients and the achievement of successful closures. Of course, counselors decided what were efficient and wise ways of managing their clients in relationship to job leads. While there was variation among counselors and from case to case (perhaps even from moment to moment), counselors managed clients in several ways: *"selling"* them to the employers, *coaching* them, *leading* them, and *avoiding damage* to their own reputations. Counselors might have used several of these strategies in managing one or more job leads for any particular client.

When employers were contacted directly concerning job possibilities, counselors stressed the capabilities of their clients, the services provided to the employers, follow-up services that would be provided (such as checking with employer and client to make sure the client was doing satisfactorily), and, where appropriate, a federal job tax credit to which they were entitled for employing the clients. In attempting to show that it was to the employer's benefit to hire their clients, counselors might turn their client's deficits into assets. For example, counselors might present a mentally retarded client's being limited to (and capable of) simple, repetitive work as an asset to an employer who wanted someone who could clean a floor and would stay at the job, not moving on or asking to move up. The thrust of the agency's marketing program was to "sell" qualified workers, not disabled individuals, to employers.

Qualified workers meant independent workers. Thus counselors were reluctant to accompany clients on interviews. To accompany a client on interviews made the "client look somewhat weak and unprepared," or it was "saying in effect that the person's so bad off that he can't even fill out an application without your [the counselor's] watching him." Instead, counselors tried to prepare clients to do well in obtaining jobs on their own (which included identifying job leads) and remaining in the jobs. One counselor explained,

> I like to try and make the person independent, to be able to fill out an application and interview on his own. You look at my R-1 notes [field notes], a lot of it's counseling towards how to interview for a job, how to look for a job. To me that's a more substantial service than finding somebody a job because that job's not going to be permanent. How many jobs are permanent? Your job isn't. Mine isn't. Something's going to change. That person is going to be a lot better off if he has knowledge that he is capable of finding a job if he has to.[4]

Whether through their own guidance and counseling or through adjustment services provided at the agency's rehabilitation center, counselors attempted to improve clients' job-seeking skills. Clients might be instructed on how to fill out an application, how to present one's disability on an application or an interview (for example, put "prefer to discuss" on an application asking if the applicant has any disability or has ever received workers compensation, and, if the subject is discussed, try to present it in a positive way, such as explaining that treatment has been received for alcoholism), what kinds of questions to expect in an interview and how to handle them, how to look for a job (for example, make a broad search rather than confining yourself to only one kind of job, or contact employers without waiting for openings to be advertised and recontact them later), and so forth.[5] Thus, just as detectives and attorneys prepare witnesses (and defendants) to do well when testifying at trials, rehabilitation counselors coached clients to prepare them for the ordeal of seeking employment.[6]

However, counselors often complained that clients were too dependent on them in managing job leads. They expected counselors to have jobs waiting especially for them. Clients who held such expectations were usually disappointed. As one counselor stated, such disappointment might lead to problematic cases:

> A lot of them [applicants] think that when they come to us there's a magic wand, and the job is going to be there because they came to us. And I don't care sometimes what you say in that initial interview, and that's one of the first things I always try to deal with is that there's no magic wand, especially the way the job market is today. I find that sometimes that reluctance, that pulling away, is because they thought that a job was going to be there automatically.

Coaching was not enough for some clients. This was true primarily for clients who, because of their disability, were unable to participate casually or competently in employment interviews, such as deaf and mentally retarded clients. For different reasons clients' inability to communicate with employers could be a great obstacle in the interviews. After perhaps "preparing" the employers for the clients and informing them they would accompany the clients, counselors interpreted for the clients and/or helped them present themselves in a favorable manner in the interviews. In varying degrees the counselors led the clients through the interviews.

In managing their clients in relation to job leads, counselors sought to avoid damaging their own and the agency's reputations with employers. Damaged reputations could jeopardize future placements. Problematic clients (those seen by counselors as possibly not "job ready" because of their "attitudes," poor work habits, failure to deal adequately with their problems such as alcoholism, and so on) could damage the counselors' and agency's reputations if counselors contacted employers on these clients' behalf and the clients did not "work out." If such clients insisted on looking for employment, then counselors might provide job leads, such as possible openings or search strategies, but they typically avoided recommending the clients to employers. If they did contact employers, they shared with them the difficulties they experienced with the clients. One counselor explained:

I'm talking about a client that has the ability to do it, but does not have the attitude to, that does not have an attitude enough to cooperate with me fully, that I cannot feel like has totally given his full effort to, and that might possibly cause the same problems, you know, to an employer. [Somebody who's missed appointments, somebody who doesn't follow through?] Somebody who has not been real cooperative. I do hesitate to make a contact and say, "I've got somebody good," when I really don't know. Now sometimes . . . these people have done fine. . . . I've given them suggestions of places to go, and they'll find employment that way and just do fine. But . . . when you make a contact, and it's a good contact, and you think that they're going to be able to hire some of your people, you've got to be real careful about some of the clients that you refer. You want to make sure that you refer them good people, that you can put your name on the line and say, "I know this particular person will work."[7]

Other human service professionals face the same problem as rehabilitation counselors: "Sticking one's neck out" for clients can damage one's ability to serve others. And other professionals may solve the problem in similar ways. As one parole officer said of a colleague who had refused to sponsor a parolee for admission to a special education program:

A PO has to be careful about who he sponsors for some of these programs. If you send a real jag down, the program might take it out on the rest of your caseload [McCleary, 1978: 97].

If human service professionals damage their reputations to those upon whom they depend when they are serving clients, then they may have served no one at all.

CATCHING CLIENTS WORKING

While counselors "ideally" should be involved actively in placing their clients—identifying job leads and managing their clients in relationship to those leads—they were not always fully involved with and aware of their clients' successes in finding work. Sometimes counselors "caught clients working."[8] While job placement activities were likely to have been undertaken, the counselors were not made aware of their clients' recent obtainment of employment. Perhaps they had had relatively little recent contact with the clients. When calling a client to determine how the client was doing, perhaps at night because previous attempts during the day were unsuccessful, a counselor might be pleasantly surprised to find that the client was working. Or, clients who had some ill feelings toward the agency and perhaps toward their counselors (for example, some former recipients of social security benefits might feel that the agency was partly responsible for their benefits being terminated) might not keep in close contact with their counselors or tell them when they found work. Through fortuitous circumstances, counselors sometimes caught the clients working. For example, when contacting nursing registries about job possibilities for her clients, one counselor happened to mention one of her clients' names and was informed that the client was working for that registry. In another case, a counselor's client

> had been "set up" as a barber by the counselor who had previously handled the caseload. The counselor received a call from the real estate agent who informed her that the client had not paid his rent for the barber shop. The counselor visited the barber shop several times but never saw the client. Sometime afterward the counselor's husband was jogging in the neighborhood, where the client also happened to live, and noticed a taxi cab in the client's driveway. The counselor later called the client, but the son said that his father was not home because he was working. The counselor finally reached the client, who claimed that he was not working. The counselor called the cab company and learned that the client was employed by the company.

After catching clients working, a counselor might provide additional services (such as counseling and guidance sessions) before closing the cases.

JUSTIFYING THE PLACEMENT

Counselors were sometimes faced with clients who obtained positions other than those developed on their IWRPs. An area administrator noted that most of the clients did not go to work in the same vocational objectives as were planned, but typically they did so within the general area that was planned. As noted in the previous chapter, counselors felt that any entry-level job would be "doing good" for clients with few skills, and, with a tight job market, even clients with skills should not be too choosy. Thus counselors might have anticipated or even encouraged clients to obtain jobs other than those listed on the IWRPs. Counselors might tell their clients to "branch out" or "look every place" to find a job.

When clients found work in areas other than those specified by the vocational objectives, counselors were required to justify that placement change. They did so with an amendment (known as an "87," the number of the form) to the plan. The 87 was used to modify not only the vocational objective but also intermediate goals, criteria, services, and length of time for the plan. One QC noted that an 87 could be a "time saver, a life saver, and many times a case saver." That was particularly true in regard to changes in vocational objectives, which could be made before as well as after the actual placement.[9]

The requirement to justify the change in vocational objectives could make the placement and successful closure that hinged on it problematic, particularly if training had been involved, according to one counselor. As another counselor declared of a case she inherited when she was assigned to a caseload:

> We have sent them [clients] to [a technical college], and they said they wanted to go into electronics. . . . I have one who is now working for the Department of Parks and Recreation, which . . . does not have any dealing with what we sent him to [technical college] for, that I'm going to have to justify. . . . He is doing well in his work, but, you know, he is not doing what we had trained him for. But with the situation as is, he explained to me, "Look, I had to get a job. This is what was available, and I have to take it." So what can you do?

What counselors tried to do was justify the change in vocational objective. However, not just any justification was acceptable. One counselor explained to me that

> he had a client whose vocational objective had been construction worker. The client could not find a job as a construction worker to which it was convenient for him to travel. Instead, the client obtained a job as a dishwasher. The counselor justified the change in vocational objective by noting that the change was convenient to the client. The justification was not accepted.

Instead, justifications needed to indicate that the changes in the vocational objectives, just like the original vocational objectives, were compatible with client's abilities and disabilities. Further, the provided services had to have an impact on the clients' obtaining their altered objectives.[10] In justifying the change, counselors might refer to the client's inability to find work in the listed objective but the availability of work in the vocation attained, the similarly between the original and present objectives (for instance, by noting the similarity of job descriptions in the *DOT*), and the related work experience of the client ("Guys in the military . . . have done a little bit of everything"). In the following case, the couselor justified, in a case development staffing group, a change to homemaker by referring to the connection between the services previously provided and the new objective:

> Due to the client's mental health problems, psychotherapy had been provided. The counselor held approximately nine "C & G" sessions with the client. The client quit her job, took a real estate course, but failed the exam to be licensed as an agent, and was now pregnant. Though the counselor suggested temporary clerical work as a possibility, the client was not interested. The counselor wondered if the vocational objective could be changed to homemaker. Perhaps the client could also attend the "homemaker program" at the rehabilitation center. The counselor explained that one area which had been worked on with the client was her being dependent and passive. The counselor wanted to help the client to become more "active," which would be useful in being a homemaker as well. The other staff members, including the QC, agreed that a change in the vocational objective would be acceptable. It was further decided that the counselor would not need to follow the client until the baby was born.

A satisfactory justification on one 87 stated:

> Client began work today as a maintenance repairer, building for [a church]. Vocational objective will be changed to maintenance repairer, building due to related military experience, his interest, and availability of employment.

CLOSING CASES

Once clients obtained employment, counselors needed to follow them for a minimum of 60 days before closing their cases as successfully rehabilitated. Follow-up was to ensure that clients were doing well when their cases were closed. According to one QC,

> It would be ideal to be able to follow him [the client] on the job, to be able to see him on the actual functioning of his job. It would be ideal to talk with one of his superiors, whether it be his immediate supervisor right on up to the manager of the place.

Some counselors did follow some of their clients in the way described above. However, in other cases, such as when the clients did not wish their employers to know of their involvement with the rehabilitation agency, phone calls and letters took the place of personal follow-up. By pretending to be a customer, one counselor even visited clients at their jobs when the clients did not want their employers to know of their involvement with the agency. For those clients caught working, particularly out of the state, follow-up was not likely to be follow-along.[11]

Timeliness was a key issue in closing cases. Successful closures were "lost" because they were not closed in a timely manner. Clients might have worked successfully for sixty days or more, but, before their cases were closed, they became unemployed. Thus counselors continually faced a dilemma in closing cases. By closing cases promptly, they were more likely to ensure a closure, but also more likely to miss clients' problems of adjustment that could jeopardize their jobs. By following cases longer, counselors might enable clients to achieve a longer-lasting rehabilitation but also risk losing some "26s." Counselors and other human service professionals face the tension that can occur between "doing good" (for the client) and "looking good" (to the agency and other observers) (Prottas, 1979: 96-97). And at times that tension might be resolved in favor of the latter.[12]

Counselors kidded each other about closing cases on the sixty-first day, particularly those they felt were "shaky." However, according to one QC, if counselors continually did that, then it would look suspicious to those who reviewed the closures. I have no information to indicate that counselors did routinely close cases that quickly, though certainly they were concerned about not losing potential 26s. Some marked on their calendars when particular cases would become eligible to be closed. One closed an expensive case while, as the counselor put it, the "closing was good":

> The agency had provided three operations for a client who had cut off his thumb in an accident. Services cost approximately $15,000. After a long period of recovery, the client obtained a job as a "night person" at a local gasoline station. However, the client had recently been involved in an armed robbery, though he claimed to have neither known that his companions in the car were planning to do the robbery nor to have been involved in the robbery. According to the client and his lawyer, it seemed that the client would receive probation. At the time of closure the client had been satisfactorily employed for more than three months and was

awaiting trial for the offense. According to the counselor, the agency had done everything which it could for the client.

Cases typically were not as dramatic as the one above. Nevertheless, counselors routinely faced the dilemma associated with closing cases. When cases were closed "quickly," counselors claimed they could always provide postemployment services to take care of any minor problem that arose, or they could open a new case if that was warranted. Counselors also realized that their need for closures sometimes prompted closing cases "when the closing was good." Some of these "quick" closures, as well as other kinds of closures, in which clients later lost their jobs, were reworked and became successful closures again. Counselors might get credit for two or more successful closures from the same client over a period of months or years. Clients "revolve through" many human service agencies' doors, not just the doors of rehabilitation or criminal justice.

In order to close a case, counselors wrote a short closure summary at the bottom of the IWRP. The summary indicated where the client was working, how much the client was earning, how and when this information was verified (verification being within two weeks of closure), that the services provided had had an impact, and that the client had been notified of the availability of postemployment services. If the counselors failed to provide the needed information in sufficient detail, such as stating that the client worked at the "main PX" without stating which military base, or if they failed to turn in the closed case within two weeks of vertification, then the mistakes had to be corrected before the area QC forwarded the case to the state office. To verify employment, counselors usually contacted the client, the client's relatives, or the employer (or a representative of the employer, such as a personnel director).[13] When contacting employers, counselors might not identify themselves as professionals with the rehabilitation agency if to do so would stigmatize their clients (who had not revealed to their employers their involvement with the agency). One closure summary read as follows:

> Planned services were provided with revision which consisted of a time extension. The client has been employed since 11/82 by [business], [city, state], [phone number], as a carpenter's helper earning $4.50 per hour, 40 hours per week. This information was verified with the client on 2/18/83. Since no further services are indicated, this case is being closed status 26, Rehabilitated. The client has been informed of impending closure and advised as to the availability of post-employment services.

MANAGING PROBLEMATIC CASES

Not all cases progressed uneventfully from the development of the IWRP to a successful closure. Many did not even become successful closures. Approximately 40 percent of the cases closed nationwide in the past several years have been closed as not rehabilitated, an increase of almost 15 percentage points during the past decade (RSA, 1983). These figures parallell those in the state I observed, except that the increase in cases closed as not rehabilitated occurred in the past half decade. When clients "got what they wanted" (such as some office visits to a doctor), failed to follow through on planned services, moved out of state, lost jobs, lost interest in finding work, failed to obtain employment, or failed to remain in contact with counselors or when counselors failed to keep in contact with clients due to oversight, large caseloads, or the cases' having been transferred from one counselor to another, then a successful closure was in jeopardy.[14]

Both the agency and counselors looked with disfavor upon unsuccessful closures. Money and time, and sometimes a great deal of both, would have been spent unfruitfully on such cases.[15] Such cases might also have led counselors to question their own professional activities and competence. As one counselor explained of problematic cases:

> Here you have spent agency money, state budget money, federal money, on this particular client, and I think it's kind of dejecting also to the counselor to know that you thought you had this person doing fine, well motivated, and then all of a sudden, "What went wrong?" Was it my fault or was it the client's fault or what?" And I think ... that ... it's something that you really sit down and try to assess. Have I done anything wrong? And I don't think that in many cases counselors particularly do anything wrong, I think once services have been provided, some clients just tend to kind of give up and say, "Hey, I got what I wanted, I really don't want to go to work."

Counselors used a variety of strategies in managing potential "28s." Among them were *contingent services, holding onto the case, tracking, persuasion, developing new angles, interpretations,* and, if all else failed, *reassigning responsibility* when closing the case as unsuccessful. These strategies were initiated by the counselor in charge of the case (though tracking was required of counselors by the agency) or suggested by fellow counselors and supervisory personnel, typically in a case development staffing. Not too surprisingly, if it seemed that their colleagues' suggestions might enable them to avoid closing a case as a 28, counselors were open to those suggestions. While counselors used these strategies in managing problematic cases, to the extent that any case was potentially problematic, counselors used them in concluding routine cases, too. Controlling cases (and clients) is a fundamental task faced by all human service professionals (Lipsky, 1980: 117-125).

Contingent Services

Counselors, particularly tough-love counselors, expected that as the agency helped the clients, the clients would help themselves. As one tough-love counselor remarked of clients, "For every action (on my part), I want a reaction (on the client's part)." Thus when counselors provided "tangibles"—medication, office visits to the doctor, transporation money to assist in looking for work—they expected clients to cooperate in following through with services and particularly in looking for work. Services were contingent upon the client's demonstration of helping themselves. Similarly, when counselors felt the agency's sponsorship of clients at a postsecondary school was problematic, they asked the clients to "go on their own" for a quarter or semester or in some other way indicate their competence and commitment. While contingent services were not always successful in enabling problematic cases to become successful closures, they did enable counselors to place some of the responsibility for rehabitation where they felt it belonged—on the clients.

Other human service professionals also tied the provision of services to their client's cooperation, commitment, and competence. As one parole officer told a "high-risk" parolee:

> Hey man, that program is expensive. You could be back in [prison] two weeks from now and all the money they spent on you would be wasted. You show me a year of good behavior on the streets and then I'll think about sponsoring you [McCleary, 1978: 97].

With the agency's recent shift in policy away from "bill paying" to substantial involvement, some counselors were concerned that it might become difficult to ensure that clients came to their offices for counseling and guidance, though others felt that if clients would not come to their offices for C and G, then they were unlikely to do well at work. In the "good old days," according to one counselor, counselors could "flavor" some counseling and guidance with work clothes (or some other desired service, such as dental work) to motivate clients to follow through. Counselors continued to use the lure of these tangibles in generating and maintaining their clients' cooperation during the delivery of services, particularly in job placement. However, if counselors were not careful enough, then they might gradually provide more services than their colleagues and superiors thought were justified and with perhaps modest movement of the client toward becoming employed. In one case that spanned several years and at least two counselors, a client who worked as a nurse and who had thrombophlebitis was bought "about eleven pair" of support hose, according to her last counselor. As the counselor who closed the case (successfully) remarked, "You know, when you go back and start checking, that's when you find this out" (that purchases had added up through the years). Without such checking and without services being contingent, their provision might not be completely successful.

Holding On

Counselors typically held onto potential 28s for months or years, generally much longer than to cases closed in status 08:

> After joining the agency and being assigned to a caseload, a counselor had seen a particular client only one time in two years. The counselor felt that the case should have been closed before she joined the agency. The client wanted the agency to sponor training as a truck driver, which the counselor explained could not be provided. The client had a bad back, which was incompatible with truck driving [and the lifting of objects into and out of truck] and had the ability to return to work as a cab driver. Phone calls and letters had not been successful in reestablishing contact with the client. However, because the counselor was now responsible for the case, she did not want to close it 28.

And at an areawide staff meeting, a QC mentioned that cases that had been opened for eight years or longer had to be closed for administrative reasons. The only question was whether to reopen them or not. According to the QC, some of the counselors were simply "postponing the inevitable." If prognosis had become poor, or if substantial services had not been provided continuously, then reopening the cases would be unlikely to lead to successful closures.

Counselors held onto cases in the hope that contact could be reestablished, that continued efforts might lead to successful placement, and/or that reluctant clients' situations would change so they would become more motivated to obtain employment. Perhaps the depletion of unemployment benefits, the conclusion of a pregancy, or the boredom of sitting at home would motivate these clients to cooperate with the counselors in finding a job. Or a client's disability, which had recently worsened, might improve.

In holding onto problematic cases, counselors not only sometimes "postponed the inevitable," but ironically and unintentionally perhaps created the inevitable. By holding onto some problematic cases for many months instead of closing them as 28s, there was little hope of doing anything constructive, according to the counselor who was recently given the responsibility of reviewing 28s and "salvaging" those that could be saved. A "new face" (that is, a new counselor) and possibly a new direction in the case could not help those cases that were "cold." However, sometimes when counselors held onto problematic cases, the cases later became successful closures. This success, as well as both the disfavor with which 28s were viewed and the service orientation of the agency, supported the strategy of holding onto cases.

Counselors not only held onto cases of uncooperative clients, but also put such cases on hold. Because counselors enjoyed working with motivated clients, believed clients could not be rehabilitated "against their will," and wanted to use their energies efficiently, at times they gave less time to clients who did not follow through with planned services. Other human service professionals may do the same (Lipsky, 1980: 152). As one tough-love counselor said of a client who told him that, because of an appointment to have her hair done, she would not be able to go to a job interview, which he "really hustled and bustled to get":

> Well, that case is still open. I didn't close it, but you can bet that I will . . . be more willing to spend them [resources] on somebody who evinces a stronger interest in getting a job. . . . Eventually I may close the case if it just becomes clear that she is disinterested in working and that was not simply a one-shot attitude on her part. . . . There are are other clients whom I could be spending my time on, and it's not fair to them to beg somebody to look for a job.

Whether counselors held onto cases or put them on hold, they hoped that by doing so they would better serve the clients and the agency.

Tracking

When holding onto cases in which contact with the clients had been lost, counselors generally tried to track the clients, particularly if they thought the clients were working. The agency required them to do so. Counselors were expected to make a personal contact, if at all possible, before closing a case as a 28.[16] And if the tracking was successful, then counselors might be able to achieve a 26 instead of a 28.

While counselors' tracking clients is not the same as detectives' locating suspects (the latter typically have more resources and greater reason to do so, as well as the threat of the law), counselors do rely on some of the strategies employed by detectives. When detectives have a suspect's name—which typically ties the person to others, such as family and friends, and to specific agencies, such as schools, businesses, clubs, and the Department of Motor Vehicles—then locating the suspect is generally not difficult. When the suspect is unknown, but an MO has been established, the detectives may use the MO to stake out a likely future target of the suspect (Sanders, 1977: 117-124). Counselors also rely on the social ties of "wayward" clients. Visits (home and otherwise), letters, contact cards, and phone calls may be made or sent to the clients, their references, and other people who know the clients (such as mental health therapists). Counselors might contact the post office in the hope of getting a forwarding address. When the federal government distributed surplus cheese in the early 1980s, some counselors used the cheese to show their appreciation to cooperative clients and to get in contact with clients who had not stayed in contact with them. If counselors thought that clients were working, they might make long-distance phone calls, sometimes even out of state calls, or make "one more try."

One way of tracking clients, making home visits, was problematic for counselors, especially, it seemed, for the female counselors. Threatening dogs, unsafe neighborhoods, dirty homes, resentful clients, suspicious family members and neighbors (Might the intruder be a bill collector or a social worker come to cut off the family's food stamps?), and wasted time were reasons some counselors did not like to do home visits, put them off, got to them when they could, had assistants do them, asked others to accompany them, and/or were glad I was along with them.[17] Home visits sometimes led counselors into foreign (even hostile?) territory. Like the "disadvantaged" clients who might have felt out of place (and therefore uncomfortable) in coming to the "middle-class bureaucracy," so some counselors felt out of place in going to their clients' homes and neighborhoods. Other human service professionals who make home and community visits, such as social workers, may have similar feelings and responses as the rehabilitation counselors (Mayer and Rosenblatt, 1975; Prottas, 1979: 31-32; Lipsky, 1980: 119-120).[18] In contrast to home visits, the significance of the professional's office became apparent.

During the course of my research, the agency instituted a trial procedure in three areas of the state that involved supervisory personnel in tracking potential 28s. The trial procedure was intended to reduce the number of unsuccessful closures, which had recently reached more than 50 percent of the number of successful closures. Supervisory personnel (a QC in the area office I observed) monitored the 28 closures as counselors turned them in. If substantial services had been provided by the agency, then the QC would try to contact the client. Through additional phoning (sometimes long distance), as well as a more thorough effort to contact references, the QC was able to contact some of these potential 28s. A few cases in which clients were contacted were closed as successfully rehabilitated (the client had been working, but the counselor had not been able to verify it) or arrangements for the agency to continue working with them were made.

The QC's efforts, particularly successes, spurred the counselors (and their assistants) to try to track their wayward clients more thoroughly. According to that QC, the counselors

> call employment service; they'll call [social service agency]. If it's a public offender, they'll even call back to the [correctional department] to see, to check . . . if the person has gone back into prison. . . . They are really doing all that they can do.

The trial procedures also spurred the counselors to obtain better references than they had in the past (for instance, not a boyfriend or girlfriend who lived with the client) and more accurate and useful information about the client's phone numbers and addresses. One counselor mentioned to me that he now photocopied the social information from the folders of applicants referred from a federal agency because that information might contain a name or phone number to use as a lead in tracking a wayward client.

The agency's trial procedure seemed to work, at least initially. During the first year in which it was employed, 28s decreased dramatically in the three test areas. They decreased to approximately two-thirds of the previous year's level, and in the local area office I studied they decreased to less than 60 percent of the previous year's level. The rest of the state decreased to only approximately 80 percent of the previous year's level.

However, the improvement was only temporary. In the next fiscal year, 28s increased dramatically in the three test offices, particularly in the area office I observed. While the rest of the state experienced a 15 percent increase in 28 closures, 28 closures increased 56 percent in the three test offices and 77 percent in the area office I observed. Almost all of the caseloads in the area office I observed experienced an increase, though some increases were much greater than others. What happened? I imagine many cases that would have been closed as 28s in the initial year of the trial program were held by the counselors. Perhaps they thought something in the clients' circumstances might change and the cases could be concluded successfully. If not, at least the counselors would be less "embarrassed" by turning in fewer 28s when there was such an emphasis to reduce them. Some counselors confirmed my hunch, though one suggested that with the new "marketing" approach, which stressed marketing-qualified workers, it would be easier for counselors to justify closing cases in status 28 by claiming that the clients would not become qualified workers. When human service professionals believe some statistic may reflect poorly on them, they may alter their behavior in order to alter those statistics (McCleary, 1978: 134). And some may just alter the statistics (Altheide and Johnson, 1980: chaps. 4, 5).

Because of the supervisor's continuing concern with the number of 28 closures and the belief that, to be effective in transforming "almost 28s" into 26s, greater attention than a QC could give was needed, the supervisor recently established a new caseload. On that caseload the counselor in charge dealt with cases that other counselors turned in as 28s. The counselor's task was to find and serve successfully as many of these clients as possible. Clients who were working (and had been served) could be closed as 26s, and others, when possible, could continue to be served. A new approach or a new face might lead to success. Even if a case did become a 28, perhaps a "better" reason for the closure could be uncovered. For instance, instead of "refusing services," perhaps the client had been institutionalized. In order to track these clients, the counselor would probably work after hours and on weekends. These problematic cases could not be handled only during regular working hours.

Persuasion

If contact had been maintained, but cooperation had not, or if contact was reestablished, then counselors were likely to try to persuade clients to cooperate in order to become successfully employed. Counselors might talk with the clients about whatever was "bothering" them or appeal to them to find jobs, either for their own sake or that of others (such as sons and daughters who could not continually provide support). Like detectives who appeal to recalcitrant witnesses' sense of civic duty (which apparently is of little use; Sanders, 1977: 106), rehabilitation counselors might appeal to clients' sense of responsibility to keep up their "end of the bargain." Counselors might ask family members and others to encourage the client to cooperate, a technique used by other human service professionals, such as parole officers. As one PO said, "Don't ever underestimate the rehabilitative power of a nagging sister" (McCleary, 1978: 112). Other counselors became more active by taking clients to appointments rather than directing the clients to them. One counselor remarked:

> I'll use anything I can to get the person interested in going to back to work, especially if I know they can or are able to go to work and should be a working member of society.[19]

Developing New Angles

Counselors might accompany persuasion with the development of a new angle on the case. A new angle might include new services to be rendered or a new vocational objective to be pursued. Counselors might send clients to the rehabilitation center for additional evaluation or adjustment services when the clients had previously failed to remain successfully in a job or benefit from services rendered, or when a new vocational objective was to be established. The counselor in charge of the recently established caseload of cases turned in as 28s believed that a new face and a new angle might occasionally prove successful. In one case, I played a very small part in possibly helping a counselor develop a new angle:

While I was in a counselor's office, she typed a rough draft of a closure summary for a case she had previously staffed to close 28. I asked the counselor to read the closure summary to me, and, in doing so, she explained the case. The client had been on the counselor's caseload since the counselor joined the agency two years ago. The client, who had diabetes, had been fired from a housekeeping position. The counselor attempted to obtain a housekeeping position for the client, but the client did not seem to be interested. Using then a personal contact, the counselor attempted to arrange for the client to work at a nursery. Learning that it was part time, the client was not interested. The counselor then arranged for the client to enter the rehabilitation center in order to determine what the client could do if she was no longer interested in housekeeping. After the first week at the workshop, the client called the counselor because the client thought that she was to be paid for her involvement at the facility. Instead, all she received was money for transportation. The counselor had previously explained to the client about reimbursement for transportation and now explained to her that during evaluation she would not earn any money unless she was involved in "contract work" (work the center contracted to do for other businesses). The client was uncertain if she wanted to return to the workshop. She did not, which the counselor learned not from her, but from the staff at the workshop. The counselor later contacted the client, who was not interested in further evaluation. At this point the counselor decided to close the case 28. After explaining the case to me, the counselor asked me what I would do. I replied that it seemed that the client was not interested in working, but I wondered if she had directly stated that. The counselor explained that when faced with job possibilities, the client claimed that she could not do that particular work. The counselor then noted that perhaps the client could keep her two granddaughters with her own daughter paying her instead of a nursery that the children currently attended. I enthusiastically endorsed that possibility.

As the above incident illustrates, the small part that I played led only to the latest angle in a series of several the counselor had already used to try to manage this problematic case.

Interpretation

In some problematic cases in which the client was working, the difficulty for the counselors was their (and others') uncertainty as to whether or not substantial services had been provided. Clients and counselors might have failed to keep in close contact; planned services might not have been completely provided (for example, only some of the scheduled psychotherapy sessions were provided); or the obtained job was "quite" different from the original objective, or perhaps was not "obviously" in line with the services rendered. Counselors, often at their colleagues' urging, might try to "see" the problematic cases as 26s rather than as 28s. As a colleague noted in one such discussion, "gummy cake [a weak 26] was better than no cake [a 28] at all." Sometimes the interpretation was successful (the QC accepted it); other times it was not. At one case development staffing,

> a counselor staffed a case where the client had been evaluated for psychological problems and had been put into plan status eight months earlier by a previous counselor. Six psychotherapy sessions were arranged, but only two were paid for. The client claimed in a recent call made to him by the present counselor that there had been "too much red tape" and that the medication he had been receiving had created unwanted side effects. The only documentation in the field notes was a summary documentation two months after the plan had been developed, which indicated that the client was "doing well" and that there were "no problems at present." Six months later the present counselor was able finally to contact the client, who had been throwing away the counselor's letters. The client was working but refused to tell where. He requested that his case be closed. The administrator (either the area supervisor or a QC) wondered if substantial services had been provided. A lengthy discussion ensued (one of the longest I witnessed) in which the present counselor in charge of the case stated that she did not know if substantial sevices had been provided, but the other counselors, while having some reservations, interpreted the "facts" as indicating that substantial services had been provided. For example, the original counselor was good at showing interest in people in the intitial interview; the client went back for a second psychotherapy session, which meant that he must have thought it was helping; the client was working and was not in a mental hospital; a "positive structure and a helping hand" had been offered; and the client would come back to the agency if he needed help (though the counselor only thought that he would). The administrator suggested that the counselor write up what had been done, and then they would "see what it look[ed] like." At the next week's staffing, the counselor, who in the meantime had contacted the client again, felt "better about a 26 now." The counselor noted that the client thanked her for the agency's help, "would definitely come back," and would refer a friend who needed help to the agency. The client provided information about his job and salary, though not his place of work. The administrator commented that he noticed that the counselor

had reservations about the case's being a 26, and that he had them, too, because it was "one of those where you could argue either way you wanted to argue. . . . It was on the line."

Whether or not a cause could be argued "either way you wanted to argue," it always had to be interpreted.

Reassigning Responsibility

If the previous strategies were not successful, then the problematic cases were closed status 28, an unsuccessful closure. When cases were closed as unsuccessful, counselors typically reassigned responsibility for the closure to other parties. I use the term "reassign" instead of "assign" because the agency and its officials made clear that counselors were responsible for their cases and the decisions made about them. Counselors were responsible for the decision to "28" a case, but when doing so they reassigned responsibility for that unwanted closure to someone else, typically the client.[20] This reassignment of responsibility was in keeping with the counselor's general attitude that clients could not be rehabilitated against their will, or, put more poetically, "You can't squeeze blood from a turnip" (see Lipsky, 1980: 152-153).

According to counselors, often 28 closures were the clients' "fault": Their medical conditions had worsened, they had left the state, they had returned to prison, they had "gotten what they wanted" and lost interest, and so forth. In some cases counselors realized that through their own and the agency's actions (for example, cases transferred from one counselor to another or counselors reassigned to different caseloads), contact with the clients had been sporadic at best. No wonder, then, that clients lost interest or failed to cooperate.

When counselors closed a case as a 28, they indicated to their colleagues and, perhaps more important, to those who would review the case later (the QC at the state level or federal auditors) that they had tried their best to serve the client, but because of the client's behavior or condition, a successful closure was not achieved. The previous strategies discussed pointed to the counselors' having done their best to serve the client. Counselors and QCs often remarked to one another that there was nothing more that could be done in the difficult case. If it were possible to have a successful 28 closure, as one QC noted, then it would be a closure in which the responsibility for avoiding that closure had been shouldered by the counselor, but responsibility for the closure itself had been the client's.

In the closure summary, counselors reassigned responsibility and through their documentation provided justification for that re-assignment. A closure summary for a 28 might look like this:

> Client has received planned services but did not follow through with scheduled counseling sessions. Numerous attempts to locate the client have been made with no success. Therefore, the case is being closed in status 28: unable to locate.

THE RECORD

While the "real" work of detectives is solving crimes, paperwork is an important, if sometimes unwanted, feature of their work. While some of it is "carried out for the sole purpose of meeting bureaucratic requirements," much of it is "done with the understanding that a good report might later prove to be important in an investigation" (Sanders 1977: 42). Paperwork, particularly documentation of what occurs during the life of a case, involves similar concerns for rehabilitation counselors and other human service professionals. It may be both a useful tool and potential trouble to be managed (Manning, 1974: 297-298; McCleary, 1978: chap. 5; Prottas, 1979: 152-153; Altheide and Johnson, 1980: chaps. 4, 5; Gubrium and Buckholdt, 1982: chap. 5).

Throughout the life of a case, rehabilitation counselors were required to document what occurred. They did so in their field notes (also referred to as the "R-1s," after the forms' identification). Docmentation could be used by counselors (or others) in serving clients, or it was addressed to bureaucratic requirements and concerns.[21] For oneself (and one's casework assistant), future counselors who might handle the case, and, infrequently, supervisory staff if counselors were not available, documentation provided a history of what had occurred in the case and an indication of where the case was (supposed to be) headed. As one QC explained to new counselors in a case manual study group, with often more than 100 cases being worked by each counselor at any time, it would be impossible to remember everything that was happening in each case. Documentation supplemented counselors' imperfect memories. With it they knew when the last contact was made with the client, what had been discussed, where the client was to look for work, and other pertinent information. When cases were transferred to a new counselor or a different counselor assumed responsibility for a caseload, the counselor's documentation enabled that counselor to develop some understanding of what had taken place in the cases. As one counselor noted of the R-1 notes of a transferred case:

> It gives you an idea . . . what that counselor was doing in addition to whether the client was cooperating, whether he was motivated, whether he was making progress. It also gives you an idea of how to deal with the client. For instance, if the client was uncooperative, then you obviously need to lay down some ground rules as soon as you see the client. If the client was demanding, then you need to know that, too. If the client . . . had a poor, let's say, contact-to-counselor ratio, in other words the counselor would try three or four times before the client would return a call or come in for a counseling session, OK, then that gives you an idea what type of person that you're dealing with.

And if the counselor in charge of the case was not available to make a decision, then the R-1 notes might help other staff members do so.

While counselors believed that documentation might enable them to serve their clients, they also realized there were other purposes for documentation. Documentation was one way of making their work visible to others. It enabled others to assess whether or not counselors were doing their job—adequately managing their cases and providing substantial services to their clients. As one QC stated, the field notes were the counselor's "tale of the service" from "day one right up to the last contact with the client prior to . . . writing up a summary for closure." However, because the QC was not present when the events occurred, if they were not documented, as far as the QC was concerned, then they did not occur—a stance taken in other human sevice agencies, such as social service agencies (Johnson, 1975: 45). Documentation was an offspring of the concern for accountability and compliance (Smits and Ledbetter, 1979). Were rehabilitation counselors and agencies, like other human service professionals and organizations, doing what they were supposed to be doing? Through documentation, counselors and agencies could be controlled.

Perhaps because of these concerns with accountability and compliance, counselors traditionally have spent a great deal of time on paperwork (almost 40 percent of their time in one study, but generally at least one-fourth of their time). Yet they have also indicated that while they would like to spend less time on paperwork, they are able to find the time to do it, even though they do not have sufficient time to carry out most of their necessary tasks (Rubin and Emener, 1979; Emener and Rubin, 1980).

Whether it was the review of a 26 closure, twice-yearly local audits, more infrequent federal audits, or other reviews, counselors' paperwork was continually being scrutinized. Documentation was done for others, but in doing it one covered oneself (and the agency) as well. Through documentation counselors could show their own and the agency's competence.[22] Through documentation counselors could protect themselves and the agency from outside criticism. Like police and parole officers, who use paperwork to protect themselves from citizens' complaints, internal investigations, challenges by other officials, or media attention (Manning, 1974; McCleary, 1978: 145-150; Gilsinan, 1982: 36-38), counselors used their R-1 notes to protect themselves from clients who might later complain they were not being served adequately. One counselor explained:

> By doing it [documentation] you're really clearing yourself because, you know, you might have a client that might get upset with you because you're not providing maybe a service that you [are] not able to provide. And you might have to say, "Well, I'm sorry, we're not able to do this." And, if you've got your R-1 documented adequately, you have no problems if that case were to be called by [the area supervisor] or somebody in the state office.
>
> [Have you ever had a case like that?]
>
> Yes, I have, I certainly have. And luckily, as I said, you know, my case was documented adequately. They could see what went on with the client, why it happened, and what I did to try to alleviate that problem.

Counselors wondered if documentation was primarily intended for others' uses, particularly federal auditors', rather than for their use in serving clients.

Doing Documentation

As one counselor noted, "No job [was] ever finished until the paperwork was done." That certainly applied to documentation. Yet when and how was it to be done? Counselors were typically responsible for more than 100 and sometimes more than 200 cases at any given time. Successive appointments, phone calls, unexpected referrals, applicants or clients, various interruptions, and the other responsibilities of managing large caseloads often made it seem to counselors that there was not enough time to do documentation. Counselors also realized that through their documentation their competence was assessed. Given the other demands they faced and the evaluative use of the R-1 notes, counselors employed various strategies in doing documentation. [23]

While counselors believed that it was best to document an event (such as a counseling session with a client) immediately after it occurred (Britten, 1981), it was not always possible to do so. The expected and unexpected demands on the counselors often led them to do documentation later, sometimes days, weeks, or even months later. Counselors might set aside some time to do their paperwork (one counselor tried to set aside one day each week to do paperwork), come in early or on the weekends to do it, take it home to be done, or get to it when they could. When counselors did not document an event immediately after it occurred, they relied on jotted notes, particularly of telephone conversations, sometimes the administrative entries made by their casework assistants on another form (where events such as the scheduling of the general medical evaluation or the return of that evaluation would be noted), and their memories. When they wrote field notes days, weeks, or months after the documented events occurred, they dated the entries to correspond with when the events occurred, not when the entries were made.

Counselors did not document everything that occurred in the life of a case. They could not have done so, nor did the agency expect them to do so. The agency's case manual stated that "since no case record will reproduce everything that is said or done in the case, the counselor is forced to be selective in what he records." According to the manual, "critical points"—such as the determination of eligibility, the client's continuing perceptions of problems, establishment of a counseling relation, the use of information (such as medical records) in the rehabilitation process, case supervision during the initial phase of training or employment of the client, and the loss of contact and efforts to reestablish contact—needed to be included in the counselors' R-1 notes.

Counselors varied widely in how much they documented, not only in how much they wrote, but in how often they wrote as well. According to one QC, counselors should have been trying to reach a happy medium, a point at which they did not become so involved in documentation that it detracted from service provision, yet they documented sufficiently to show substantial services had been provided. Some counselors "confessed" that they were perhaps "too wordy"; others attempted to be very succinct:

> I summarize a lot. I give you the example: If a client comes in here and I talk to him about his appearance, his shirt, the color of his shirt that doesn't match with the pants, his unkempt appearance, shoes, . . . his face . . . not washed, stuff like that. My documentation would be brief— "counsel client about his appearance and about being ready for a job," period. Another counselor might elaborate that in half a page. But I don't, I don't have that kind of time.

However, counselors could also be too succinct. According to one QC, entries such as "saw client today—provided guidance and counseling" were not detailed enough to show the counselor's substantial involvement in the case. Sufficient and complete documentation has been seen as a problem in rehabilitation agencies (Rubin, 1977).

Counselors did not document every contact with their clients, though some documented more than others. Counselors were unlikely to document, for instance, when a client called to check on whether or not his or her medical examination had been scheduled or if the results had been received. Instead, counseling sessions (even if only lasting several minutes over the phone), reviews of pertinent information (such as psychological reports), development of the IWRP, service provision, and other (critical) events that seemed to relate to the progress of the case and the counselor's involvement in it were documented. Some counselors documented single contacts and events. Others relied more heavily on "summary" entries, in which they documented what had transpired in the case since the previous entry, which might have been several months ago. The continued use of summary entries, each covering several months in the life of the case, might be criticized by a QC or by federal auditors for not adequately documenting consistent counselor involvement.

I had few occasions in which I observed both an activity involving a counselor and the counselor's documentation of that activity. Numerous comparisons between the actual activity and the entry in the R-1 notes would be needed to begin to develop an in-depth understanding of that part of doing documentation. However, it was clear to me that in their documentation counselors constructed an account of what transpired during the life of a case. They did not provide a literal account. A microanalysis of how counselors construct entries must wait for other investigations.

Because documentation was a selective construction of what took place during a case, it had less meaning for others than for the counselor who wrote it (see Gubrium and Buckholdt, 1982: 148). When counselors reviewed their field notes, the entries brought to mind additional information concerning the event. That did not happen to naive readers, such as auditors, QCs, and counselors to whom the case had been transferred. In part, this was the cause for the tension between writing enough in the R-1s to show involvement, but not so much that clients were neglected. What was enough for knowledgeable readers (that is, the counselors involved) may not have been enough for naive readers. Similarly, when detectives read old reports for investigative purposes, they often need to be "filled in" by someone who is familiar with the events documented in the report (Sanders, 1977: 65).

I asked one counselor to read an R-1 entry and then (briefly) explain what had occurred during the event entered in the field notes. The entry appears below, followed by the explanation:

> Met with client to sign IWRP. Counseled him on appropriate job-seeking behavior. Gave him a long list of places to contact. Encouraged client to maintain contact with counselor.

> That's one entry, and that was an hour. Okay. We sat down. We pulled out the phone book. We made a list of places to contact. We talked about transportation. We talked about how to dress when we go on interviews. We talked about motivation, getting up off his rear-end and going. You know, we talked about *all* that stuff, and he walked out of here with a list of places and phone numbers. We talked about whether or not it would be better to go in person or to call. We talked about going over to where he used to work and getting a letter of recommendation. We talked about all that stuff. Which is stuff that he really couldn't do for himself [your average human being could], but, because of his disability, just doesn't have the initiative to do that on his own. So, but, that right there proved that I was doing my job for that client.

Perhaps a microanalysis is not needed in light of the above-cited counselor's last statement. As long as counselors' documentation showed (to others' satisfaction) that they were doing their job, then (given that their documentation was not a fabrication) the detailed relationship between what they wrote and what took place may have been relatively unimportant to all concerned.

TREATING THE RECORD

In order to show they were doing their job, counselors "treated the record." Once, when I accompanied a counselor in the field, the counselor commented that instead of stating in their field notes that they "talked" with their clients, counselors typically recorded that they "counseled" their clients. In criticizing staff who were more concerned with numbers and "looking good" than with serving people, this counselor called the above and similar uses of language "treating the record." I use the term without that intended criticism. Counselors not only had to treat (serve) clients, they also had to treat paperwork. Counselors needed to do both competently in order to be successful. Even the best counselors knew that it was through their documentation that their competence was known and shown to others, especially far-away others, such as federal auditors. If those others viewed the documentation as inadequate, then they were likely to question the adequacy of services rendered and the competence of the counselors. Counselors still varied widely in their styles of documentation; some documentation was evaluated by QCs and others as more adequate than other documentation. But whether their documentation was more or less adequate, or even inadequate, counselors "treated the record" (among other things) when they did documentation.[24]

Counselors "treated the record" when they recorded in their field notes that they "counseled" with their clients. Because "C and G" was an essential service that counselors provided to all clients, it needed to be recorded in an appropriate way. "Talk" would not do. When counselors used summary entries instead of no entries at all, dated those entries according to when the events occurred rather than when the entries were made, and divided one summary entry into two or more in order to show consistent counselor involvement, they were treating the record. When counselors recorded that the IWRPs were developed by them and their clients because QCs, auditors, and others who reviewed the field notes "liked" such statements, then counselors had treated the record (and had done so even though the clients were involved, as they typically were, in the development of their IWRPs). When counselors made an addition or correction to an entry, because otherwise a reviewer might not have realized that substantial services were provided (for example, if a counselor did not merely take a client to an interview, but counseled with the client beforehand) or the reviewer might have misunderstood what occurred, then counselors were treating the record. When counselors systematically attempted to "catch up" with their documentation, either by contacting applicants and clients who had not kept in contact or by making entries in the field notes of past contacts so that there would not be gaps longer than two to three months in the documentation (and hence in the rehabilitation process), they were treating the record (see Chapter 5).[25] When QCs allowed counselors to document unrecorded contacts with clients in order to show that substantial services had been provided in 26 closures and counselors did so, the record had been treated. Anytime counselors were documenting for others and not for themselves (even when done honestly, as I imagine was usually the case), they were treating the record. The record (and others who might review it) was being directly "served," not the clients. Often when human service professionals do paperwork, they are treating the record (Altheide and Johnson, 1980: chaps. 4, 5; Gubrium and Buckholdt, 1982: 145-148).

Because counselors varied greatly in their documentation, it is difficult to speak of a typical set of R-1 notes. Below is one set of R-1 notes that was not unusual. Entries were typed and/or handwritten. Each was initialed by the staff member who wrote it, typically the counselor, though at times a casework assistant or other staff member might write an entry. Initials or signatures, also used in other human service agencies, such as parole agencies (McCleary, 1978: 131), aid in the quest for accountability. Abbreviations ("clt" for "client," for instance) were often used, but for the sake of clarity I have not kept the abbreviations. Depending on the case and the counselor, other field notes would be more or less lengthy and greater or fewer in number. Some of the information has been rephrased or deleted so that the counselor and client cannot be identified. The case itself has proceeded relatively quickly. Most would not be worked and concluded in a few months. If no problems occurred in the future, then the case could have been closed as a successful rehabilitation approximately three months after it was opened.

2/23/82   Survey interview. Client is a 27-year-old single male. Currently on psychiatric care at [name] Hospital for depression. Has history of several admissions. Has not worked since left army in August '80. Does not know what he really wants to do. I counseled him about workshop. . . . Client says he wants to work. He seemed alert and oriented today. He may be a good candidate for training. Is probably above-average intelligence. Will get medical records.

2/23/82   Received records. Diagnosis—depression over the past two years. Goals of last hospitalization not accomplished. Dissatisfied with self and walking off and avoiding responsibility.

3/2/82   Saw and counseled with client at [name] Hospital. We spoke about possible training. Maybe staying at [name of halfway house for individuals with mental health problems]. Will be discharged in about one week. According to nurse is sleeping okay and behaving appropriately. Would likely be good candidate for training. I counseled him about [technical college] . . . etc.

3/9/82   I counseled with client at [hospital]. He seems to be more interested in job now. Will likely stay at [halfway house] upon discharge. . . . I counseled him about job hunting. He has a job interview at [name of business] tommorrow. He has also been referred to Job Service. I am going to counsel next week if he is interested in a job. I will proceed with IWRP.

3/12/82   CDS concurs with IWRP for treatment at [name] Hospital, counseling and guidance, job placementd assistance and follow-up. [This entry, which is routine on R-1 notes, was initialed by the casework assistant who attended the staffing to record such information.]

3/16/82   Saw and counseled with client at [name] Hospital. He definitely wants a job and will live at [halfway house] when discharged. Probably 3/23. I counseled him about jobs. He is to visit movie theater regarding job as a projectionist. Also has interview with nursing home for job as an orderly. Also will visit [fast food restaurant] for possible job. I will assist with placement. Job at [company] requires experience. I feel [client's name] is a good candidate for job placement. Counseling will continue.

3/23/82   Saw and counseled with client at [name] Hospital.Discharged today into [halfway house] to live. Client has second interview today at [fast food restaurant] on [address]. I counseled him about interview techniques. He is to contact me regarding results of job interview.

3/24/83   Client called. Has job at [fast food restaurant]. Starts today at 4 o'clock. Will let me know salary and hours when sure. I will visit on the job.

3/30/83   Staffed case with [official] at [hospital]. Client apparently doing well at [halfway house] and on new job. Called [halfway house] left message.

CONCLUSION

Unlike detectives, who have typically done their job when they have "made a case" against suspects, rehabilitation counselors and other human service professionals have not yet done their job when they have "made a case" for clients. Once a case has been made, counselors and other human service professionals serve the clients in order to change them. They continue to work the cases in order to conclude them.

In concluding cases, rehabilitation counselors attempted to identify job leads and manage their clients in relation to those leads. They did so in order to place them. Once clients were placed and satisfactorily employed, couselors closed their cases. Yet not all cases proceeded uneventfully. Counselors often managed problematic cases. However, to the extent that all cases were potentially problematic until they were (successfully) concluded, the strategies used by counselors in managing problematic cases were the strategies used (in modified form, perhaps) to conclude any case. And, ironically, it was in the record that, for many people, the case came to life.

If counselors were successful in concluding a case, then they (and the agency) received credit for another 26, much like detectives, who receive credit for another "collar" or clearance when they are successful in working a case. However, just as the clearance of a crime fails to disclose the activities that went into its production, so the 26 closure fails to reveal the activities that went into its creation. While to a great (but also changing) extent the agency saw one 26 as the same as another 26, the counselors' activities may have been greatly different from one 26 to another. "Hard" data often become much "softer" when what goes into their production is examined more closely (Gubrium and Buckholdt, 1979; Bogdan and Ksander, 1980). And in producing those 26s and other closures, counselors did not merely handle individual cases, they managed a large number of cases. They managed caseloads.

NOTES

1. After detectives have made a case, their job may not be completely done. In rape cases they may work closely with the prosecuting attorney's office in "coordinating a strategy for prosection" and in being "responsible for supporting the victim during the trial period" (Sanders, 1980: 109). However, more investigation is needed of what detectives do after they have "made a case."

2. The ambivalence among counselors is paralleled by the great amount of discussion, often conflicting, among rehabilitation educators and professionals concerning various aspects of placement, such as its nature, what it entails, the philosophy behind it, and the broad orientation to use, not to mention the specific strategies to employ or not to employ (Zadny and James, 1976; Salomone and Usdane, 1977; Usdane and Salomone, 1977; Wright, 1980: Sect. V; Olshansky, 1981; Vandergroot, 1981).

3. Counselors in the West reported that clients, the employment service, want ads, and employers contacted during job development work were the four most frequent ways of identifying job leads. Counselors reported using different strategies for identifying job leads (actually methods of obtaining jobs) depending on whether clients were severely disabled or not. When working with severely disabled clients, counselors were more likely to depend on employers who previously had hired clients and on job orders placed with the

agency. "Evidently, working with the severely disabled led counselors to seek out placements where their clients would have better-than-average chance of succeeding" (Zadny and James, 1979a: 371). The "formal" leads, such as want ads and the employment service, tend to be unproductive but are also overused, perhaps because of their convenience (Zadny and James, 1977a, 1978). In professional journals counselors' colleagues provide tips on how to identify job leads (Britten, 1981). One tip is to use obituary notices, which is "only used in extreme desperation or as a tour de force by the accomplished placement strategist" (Flanagan, 1974: 212).

4. Counselors in the West seem to share a similar sentiment, crediting more than half of the successful placements to clients and less than one-third to themselves. Equivocal findings suggest that client job seeking may be more productive than counselor intervention, although counselor contact with employers was related to various caseload measures of successful rehabilitation (Zadny and James, 1979a).

5. See Wright (1980: 654) for advice to counselors on how to counsel clients about disclosing their disabilities. Given the discrimination against those with disabilities (Link, 1982), discretion (or is it deception?) may be the better part of wisdom in clients' disclosing their disabilities and counselors' advising clients how to do so. Counselors believed that "full disclosure" was not always the best policy for the clients.

6. Such coaching, however, may not have a great impact on counselors' placement rates (Zadny and James, 1979a: 366-367).

7. With the recognition that present clients can influence future placement opportunities with an employer, one rehabilitation professional advises agencies to select "model" clients when initially contacting an employer (Wright, 1980: 668).

8. Perhaps half of rehabilitated clients find jobs on their own, though "on their own" may involve leads and suggestions from the counselors and other rehabilitation professionals (Zadny and James, 1977a; Wright, 1980: 646). Only in some of these cases, however, have counselors caught clients working.

9. A study of clients placed in several western states and territories revealed that either there was a "consistent pattern from occupation at original plan to occupation at closure" or there was "no congruency between the planned occupational training and the occupation at closure" (Rubin, 1975: 375). Perhaps in many of these latter cases counselors caught clients working in jobs that were incongruent with the orginial vocational objectives and then, where necessary, justified the placement changes before closing the cases.

10. For a discussion among rehabilitation professionals about the congruence between vocational objectives and attainments, see Bowman and Micek (1973), Rubin (1975, 1977), and Zadny and James (1976). A GAO (1982: 11) audit reported that in about 35 percent of the status 26 closures reviewed in five states there was

no apparent relationship between the clients' jobs at case closure and the vocational rehabilitation services provided. In some cases, counselors established clients' vocational goals after clients had found employment or changed clients' goals to show closer matches between training services and job placement. In other cases, counselors closed client's cases as homemakers when clients did not fulfill their vocational plans.

The GAO concluded that the accomplishments of vocational rehabilitation agencies were overstated.

11. Follow-up activities did not seem to be related to measures of rehabilitation productivity or the nature of closures within several western states in the mid-1970s (Zadny and James, 1979a).

12. From 1972 to 1975, in Alaska one-third of rehabilitated cases were closed during the first month they were eligible for closure. The investigators "doubt that even a bare majority of cases nationally are closed during the first month eligible for closure" (Zadny and James, 1976: 60). Such information suggests that if counselors are concerned about closing cases quickly, that concern is managed along with other concerns and contingencies that work against closing cases as soon as they are eligible for closure.

13. In one case, a counselor used a friend, "really a lover," in order to verify employment. That was "probably the most uncomfortable" verification the counselor had done. Another counselor remarked wistfully to some of his colleagues that six or seven years ago a case could be closed if a mother was contacted and she said that her daughter was working, but she did not know where. A counselor's word was honored. Today, that would not be adequate verification. A third counselor, after having "dragged" out of a client where she was working, confirmed that she was employed but not obtaining a salary and, having made several previous phone calls, the counselor decided to list her salary as $3.35 per hour, minimum wage. The counselor did not think the client could have been "making all that much money" because she was a part-time clerk.

14. In a recent fiscal year, approximately 23 percent of the status 28 closures in the agency I observed were due to the counselor's inability to contact or locate the client or the client had moved, 26 percent to the client's failure to cooperate, 18 percent to the client's refusal of further services, 12 percent to unfavorable medical prognoses or handicaps that were too severe, 11 percent to the client's institutionalization, 3 percent to the clients' death or transfer to another agency, and 8 percent were "other."

15. In the first six months of a recent fiscal year in the agency I observed, the average cost for case services (such as prostheses, medical follow-up, and the like, but *not* salaries or overhead) was approximately $450 for successful closures and $300 for unsuccessful closures. These figures would be likely to be much higher in other states that purchase many services provided "in-house" by the rehabilitation centers of the agency I observed. Unsuccessful closures cost this agency more than $1 million in recent years, a figure that would be much higher if salaries and overhead were taken into account.

16. The agency required its counselors to try to contact clients personally before closing their cases 28, in order to avoid cases such as the following, which occurred in another state:

> A 17-year-old man, disabled by severe asthma, was referred to the . . . Division of Vocational Rehabilitation. The client's asthmatic condition required that he avoid working in humid or dusty conditions or where there would be sudden temperature changes. His plan for rehabilitation included financial assistance in becoming a commercial artist through a community college. However, the client did not enter school but obtained work on a . . . freighter. This work apparently aggravated his asthma, and he had to be hospitalized. The case was closed as unsuccessful at that point without contacting the client, because the client "failed to cooperate." The case file contained a report from a psychologist, prepared early in the rehabilitation process, indicating possible personality problems. We believe, and State officials concurred, that these problems should have been explored and that the client should have been contacted before his case was closed to determine why he had not entered college [GAO, 1973; 27].

17. In making home visits (and on other occasions), some counselors used deception. Counselors, like detectives (Sanders, 1977: 105-106), may be faced with reluctant people who may have valuable information. Though I observed no instances of deception,

counselors sometimes advised others to use it or spoke of others who in the past had done so. For example, when making a home visit to contact a client, especially if cooperation from family and friends had not been forthcoming, some counselors might claim (or were advised to claim) that they had a check for the client or an unpaid bill from the hospital that if not paid, might lead others to track down the client.

18. Home visits and other trips out of the office also enabled counselors to conduct personal business, such as banking and shopping. Counselors were required to log out and log in when leaving and returning to their offices. If necessary and possible, the logs would enable the agency to contact counselors in the field or at least to know when counselors would return.

19. See Wright (1980: 522-525) for a discussion of clients' motivation problems and solutions to those problems.

20. In status 28 closures in which cases had been transferred to counselors from other area offices, but counselors had never been able to contact the clients, the counselors would reassign responsibility to the counselors formerly in charge. As one counselor who received such cases remarked, "When it [the 28 closure summary] is written up, I just spill my guts and tell them, 'I've never seen the client. The case was transferred in.'" These cases suggest that some counselors handle problematic cases by bureaucratically reassigning responsibility (that is, transferring the cases) to other counselors, a practice also used by parole officers, who may send troublesome clients to special treatment programs in order to get rid of them (McCleary, 1978: 141-144).

21. According to the case manual, case recording had three purposes: to facilitate the evaluation of the client by bringing together pertinent information; to improve staff and agency evaluation, in-service training, research, and other services; and to ensure that the programs of the agency met criteria set by law and regulations. See Wright (1980: 601) for ten critical uses of case recording.

22. To some rehabilitation professionals, "good case-recording is probably highly correlated with good casework," and the "well-qualified counselor takes pride in the record as a documentation of skill and devotion" (Wright, 1980: 600). The counselors I observed viewed case recording in a different and more complex way than the above statement suggests.

23. See Wright (1980: 601-604) for some problems in and principles for case recording.

24. See McCleary (1978: 57-60, chap. 5) for a discussion of parole officers and paperwork. POs don't do paperwork only to show their competence to others. They also use records to do their work: to threaten parolees, get rid of troublesome parolees, and protect themselves and the agency.

25. The paperwork requirements encountered by human service professionals, such as social workers, may serve to

> reverse what one might think to be the expected relationship between the actual social service activities and the reports. [The] prospect of an impending record or report stimulate[s] provision of service. Thus, an approaching deadline for completion of a report on one's actions often serves [s] as justification for a visit to the home of a welfare client even though it [is] not necessary [Johnson, 1975: 45].

5

MANAGING CASELOADS

During the course of a day, detective work "consists of a mosaic of little tasks," such as reading reports, looking for suspects, establishing crimes, going to court, catching up on paperwork, and making contacts (Sanders, 1977: 128). Each day, detectives may be handling many cases. While concluding the investigation on some, they are likely to receive new reports on others. They manage a mix of cases that they have worked to various stages in the investigative process. For example, in one sheriff's department on the West Coast, a detective in the juvenile detail handled more than 100 cases in a 12-week period, though many received "minimal investigative attention" (Sanders 1977: 133-134). Therefore, to understand detective work, one must understand not only how detectives work individual cases and conduct specific investigations, but also how they organize their efforts in dealing with many cases. This is particularly important for rehabilitation counselors and other human service professionals.

Rehabilitation counselors, like other human service professionals, have responsibility for many cases at the same time (Zimmerman, 1966: 257-261). In the course of a day, counselors may see several referrals, develop an IWRP, counsel a client, review medical records, and talk with an employer. They handle a mix of cases that are at different stages in the rehabilitation process and that may require different responses. In the office I investigated, rehabilitation counselors routinely managed more than 100 cases at a time, and more than 200 in the recent past. Counselors did not just work and conclude individual cases, they handled many cases simultaneously; they managed caseloads.

Counselors' concerns in managing their caseloads transcended the management of individual cases. They were assigned responsibility for caseloads. Goals were set for their caseloads. Their caseloads were audited. They behaved in ways that clearly spoke to a concern greater than that given to any individual case, such as attempting to avoid damage to their reputations when placing clients. Of course, caseloads did involve many individual cases. Counselors juggled the demands of 100 or more cases in attempting to serve each individual. I imagine that, without caseload concerns, counselors would have handled individual cases quite differently at times. Yet individual cases were not all counselors handled when they managed caseloads (Wright, 1980: 170-174; Cox et al., 1981).

To have caseloads, counselors had to have individual cases with which to work. They needed to *manage referrals,* which consisted of both developing and working referral sources. But, faced with hundreds of cases during the course of a year, and typically more than 100 cases at any time, counselors also needed to manage their activities. They *organized their work.* In doing so, the *pace* of their caseloads and the cases they contained was an important concern to them. And in working and concluding cases, as well as in managing their caseloads, counselors were involved in *staffings,* a prominent feature of human service work.

MANAGING REFERRALS

Without crimes to solve, detectives would be out of work. Without clients to serve, rehabilitation counselors and other human service professionals would also be unemployed. Detectives typically wait for possible crimes to be brought to their attention by patrol officers. With the general exception of vice and narcotics officers, detectives are *reactive* in their work (Sanders, 1977: 48-52). They react to the field reports of patrol officers, who have themselves reacted to the complaints of citizens. Rehabilitation counselors tend to be much more *proactive* in their work. In comparison to detectives, they are more likely to seek out potential clients to serve. As one counselor remarked, "I think you really have to advertise and go out and seek referrals. You can't just sit here all day and expect them to come in." Other human service professionals may also be proactive at times, such as social workers who "reach out" to recruit clients for various programs (Altheide and Johnson, 1980: 145) or drug abuse workers in a fee-for-service or reimbursement arrangement who attempt to "drum up business" due to a lack of demand (Peyrot, 1982: 166).[1]

Rehabilitation counselors must be relatively proactive because citizens may not realize that they have potentially significant impairments; if they do, they may not know where to go, or, if they know, they may be reluctant to go. Citizens have relatively little familiarity with vocational rehabilitation agencies, so relatively few who might benefit from its services apply on their own (Haug and Sussman, 1968: Sussman et al., 1969; Williams and Edwards, 1971; Haug et al., 1974; Wright, 1980: 230).[2] In contrast, detectives can be more reactive because citizens have a fairly good understanding of what constitutes crime (Gibbs and Erickson, 1979), and they know that police are officially authorized to deal with crime. When there are relatively few victims or complainants, such as in vice and narcotic offenses, detectives become more proactive.

Consequently, the rehabilitation agency and its counselors were concerned with increasing the public's awareness about their potential for being served by the agency. The agency attempted to increase the public's awareness through publicity: stories in the news media, brochures and reports, awards, and so forth. The counselors' immediate concern was referrals.

Without referrals, counselors had no cases to work. The case manual stated that the "first basic principle necessary to the successful operation of a vocational rehabilitation program is the establishment and development of a well-organized system of referrals." Counselors recognized this principle. Therefore, they were concerned about obtaining enough referrals and that their sources did not "dry up."

The importance of and concern with referrals among the staff became apparent in the adjustment of territories and referral sources. One counselor who obtained more referrals yearly than anyone was required several times to share his referral sources with others. The significance of referrals appeared in the friendly kidding among counselors concerning "stealing" one another's referrals. Among counselors who shared referral sources, if one was absent, then a referral who was usually directed to the absent counselor might be directed to the other. This friendly kidding, however, pointed to the underlying competition that could exist among counselors. As one counselor noted:

Well, I'm going to let the cat out of the . . . bag, and I say that because whenever you're dealing with referral sources, naturally, if you get referrals, that means somebody else is less likely to. So there's some competition, which probably is helpful and healthy. Otherwise, people would sit back and do nothing.

Most counselors could not afford to "sit back and do nothing." Had they done so, they would have soon been out of referrals and ultimately out of a job.

Referral sources varied. As the case manual stated, counselors "must depend to a very large degree upon the fullest cooperation of interested individuals and agencies to refer disabled persons" to them. The manual provided examples of a wide variety of referral sources, including the American Cancer Society, artificial appliance companies, doctors, employers, hospitals, interested individuals, religious organizations, schools, social services departments, and the Veterans Administration. Counselors developed and worked these and other referral sources to obtain potential clients to serve.

DEVELOPING REFERRALS

Counselors typically worked referral sources that were already established. During the course of my research, however, I learned about some relatively recently developed referral sources and observed some efforts by counselors to develop referrals in two small, out-of-the-way communities that had not been served systematically in the past. In developing referrals, counselors needed to "sell" the agency and themselves to others so potential clients would learn about and contact the agency.[3] To do that, counselors first had to identify potential referral sources. Likewise, narcotics detectives need to identify and develop informants if they are to control the narcotics trade (Skolnick, 1966: chap. 6).

Counselors identified potential referral sources through happenstance and through a more systematic examination of possibilities. Through a chance encounter with a fellow patron of a local nightclub, one counselor identified a referral source. The patron worked at a health agency, which later became a referral source for the counselor. Another counselor bumped into a federal rehabilitation professional, who mentioned to the counselor that he could use some help with patients in an addiction and treatment unit at a local Veterans Administration hospital. A very successful referral source developed from that chance encounter.

Counselors also identified potential referral sources in a more systematic manner. A counselor who served hearing impaired clients contacted administrators of a local school district and later made a presentation to the teacher and students in a high school program for hearing-impaired youth. Letters were sent to parents to notify them of the availability of rehabilitation services for their children. Another counselor, upon being assigned a new territory, decided to contact a large military installation located within the territory:

> I looked up in the telephone book and said, "What do they have out at Fort [name]?" . . . I saw the chaplain. So I called the chaplain and I said, "Here's what we do. Whom can I speak with out there to reach some of the dependents of Fort [name]?" It just came to me. He said, "Well, I don't know. Why don't you try Army Community Service?" So I went over there, I got an appointment, I talked with the people, and they were very impressed with what we could do. They thought that a lot of people could utilize our service. They suggested that I contact the leader of the Fort [name] newspaper, which I did, and last Friday I got an interview with them. So in the next couple of weeks VR will be advertised, in a sense, through that interview with me. There's a referral source that really had never been tapped. And now it will be.

For that referral source to be tapped, the counselor developed it further. The counselor

> talked with a major in charge of the Social Services Department at the base hospital, explaining to the major how the rehabilitation agency could benefit the military installation. The counselor was invited to come to the discharge meetings at the hospital, although the major did not believe that the counselor would want to come every time. However, the counselor did. The counselor learned about the separate psychiatric ward at the hospital and got a "foot in that door" through use of the name of the major in the Social Services Department. After learning about the outpatient mental health clinic and being "brushed off" by a sergeant at the clinic, the counselor "went over his head" to the major in charge of psychiatric services. The major was furious that the counselor had been "slapped in the face." Since then the counselor and spouse have been invited to parties at the base, and the counselor has become a "regular member of the crew."

In the two small, out-of-the-way communities, counselors developed referrals in several ways. These communities previously had not been worked systematically. Officials at the high schools in both communities were contacted. They served as referral sources for students and were asked to spread the word among the adults of the communities. Counselors gave their business cards to adults who contacted them. The adults were asked to distribute them to friends who might need services and wanted to work. Posters informing the citizens about vocational rehabilitation were placed in prominent places around each town, such as the high school, post office, town hall, restaurants, and grocery stores. The posters stated simply:

> If you are unable to work because of a disability, contact your local vocational rehabilitation office.

Beneath that message was the name of the counselor, a telephone number, and a place, time, and date where the counselor could be contacted. Mayors and other well-known citizens were contacted. All this was done to make the communities aware of the vocational rehabilitation program.

Months later one counselor remarked of the small community he had developed:

> I'm real pleased. My adults are picking up. For the last three weeks I've had three or four people there to see that had scheduled appointments there with the school to see me.... The winter was slow, and it really has 't started picking up until just recently.... It takes a while, and then [town's name] is just such a small area that you're not going to, you can't expect to go to [town's name] and get, you know ... eight or nine [referrals] every week, every time you go.

> [Right, it's going to be hopefully a good referral source, but a small one?]

> A small one and a very slow one.

WORKING REFERRALS

Once counselors developed referral sources, they worked them. While relatively few counselors had much experience in developing new referral sources, all counselors worked their present sources. As one counselor explained about referral sources:

> Some will pan out, some won't. Some of it is luck because of the kinds of people you end up meeting. If the person at the referral source ... is tired

of his job and just marking time, he's going to be less enthusiastic about what he's doing because what does he care, it's not going to give him.... Unfortunately, we can't reimburse referral sources a dollar a referral or something. I wish we could. I think it would be a very good use of funds if we could give a referral source a dollar for every good referral we get. Unfortunately that would not be legitimate. So you have to somehow constantly market what you're doing to get these people to want to refer to you where there's no vested interest on their part.

In working referral sources so they might pan out, counselors *constructively socialized* with the referral sources, *served the sources,* and attempted to *maintain professional relations* with them. Some counselors were more successful than others.

In working referral sources, counselors were not "all business," though part of their "constructive socializing" (a term used by one counselor) was "good business." Informal conversations, shared lunches, overlooking a source's "peculiarities," putting up with sexist jokes, and the like enabled counselors to maintain cordial relations with their referral sources. As the counselor quoted above explained:

> If for some reason there was a hiatus [between seeing clients at another human service agency], I would go back to the referral sources [at that agency] and make contacts. You can't always go and keep selling your case, people just get tired of you. So you have to do a certain amount of constructive socializing, too. "Hey, how's it going?" ... You tell a joke, they laugh. They tell you one.... Then they say, "Oh by the way, I've been working with a guy that blah, blah, blah, and here's his name. Why don't you give him a call?"

While in the field (that is, seeing people in the community), another counselor stopped at a human service agency where she had once worked. She chatted with several former colleagues and showed them pictures of her family. She did this, in part, so that her former colleagues would continue to think of her when they had clients who might be served appropriately by the vocational rehabilitation agency. Similarly, detectives may use first names with their informants, be sympathetic, or at least nonjudgmental, about their informants' addictions (or criminal conduct), inquire about their health, and in other ways develop a civil relationship with those who are otherwise often despised (Skolnick, 1966: 130-132).

Detectives also provide inducements to informants so they will inform. Through reduced charges and other "breaks" (which rest on the threat not to provide them), varying amounts of money, and "dignifying the character" of the informant, detectives develop the cooperation of informants. Informants repay that kindness with information about crimes and criminals (Skolnick, 1966: 124-132).

Similarly, counselors attempted to serve their sources in some way. By doing so, sources saw the advantage of working with the counselors. As one counselor put it, "We scratch each other's backs." This might include being listed on a disabled student's IEP (individualized educational program, a recent federal requirement similar to an IWRP). It might include placing these student clients in jobs. While this was part of the counselor's responsibilities, placement showed the school officials that the vocational rehabilitation program could help them greatly in serving their students. Another counselor served his referral source by working with an employee of a private company. The counselor's referral source provided assistance to "troubled" employees of government agencies and private businesses that contracted with the referral source. Again, while the counselor's involvement with the employee was part of the counselor's responsibilities to serve eligible individuals, that involvement could be used by the referral source when contacting the employer to "sign up" the employer for services. By effectively providing services to clients that were not provided by the referral sources themselves, counselors were serving their sources as well as the clients.

In serving their sources, counselors might accept "bad" cases in which it was very doubtful, if not hopeless, that the applicants could be served successfully. They did so to maintain good relations with the referral sources. As one counselor noted of a school-age client he felt was not likely to be successfully rehabilitated, "You have to take a lot of these, you know. You have to take a lot of these in order to get the other referrals from the school."

When counselors were developing a referral source initially, some might be especially likely to accept "bad" cases. However, not all the rehabilitation professionals in the office agreed with this practice. Instead of viewing the acceptance of "bad" cases as "PR work" used to develop a solid relationship with a new referral source or maintain a good relationship with an established referral source, the critics characterized such practice as "poor screening" of referrals.[4]

Finally, counselors attempted to maintain professional relations with their referral sources. To do so, counselors typically scheduled regular contacts with the referral sources, particularly with human service agencies or outlying communities to which the counselors traveled, instead of the communities' citizens coming to the counselors. Many counselors scheduled specific times, usually weekly, to visit mental health centers, hospitals, drug abuse centers, schools, and other agencies to pick up referrals as well as work with those who had already been contacted. Counselors who appeared erratically were not particularly successful in picking up referrals. Counselors were also advised to inform, and some told me they tried to inform, their referral sources of what action they took on each referral.

To maintain professional relations, counselors also educated referral sources as to who would be likely candidates for the agency's services. The case manual stated:

> The continuous training of the referral agencies as to the types of cases acceptable for VR services will tend to reduce the time spent in screening prospective clients.

While some supervisory personnel and counselors stated that it was best for referral sources, particularly human service agencies such as mental health clinics, which served people with some kind of problem, to refer everybody so the counselors could do their own screening, often that was not done. When counselors initially developed referral sources, they educated them about the agency and its services. When policy changes occurred, as they did regarding the agency's provision of substantial services instead of "bill paying," referral sources might be reeducated. Doctors were informed of such changes. New professionals at a referral source might be educated when they sent "nearly everybody." The acceptance and rejection of referrals was an indirect way of educating referral sources as to who should or should not be referred.

Just as counselors typically opened cases on those who wanted to work and, with services, were likely to work, so might they educate their referrals to send them such people. In explaining what was told to professionals at one human service agency, a counselor stated:

> I try to tell them, you know, send people to me that had worked in the past and had pretty good work history when they worked, and like if they maintained a job for more than six months. Don't send me someone that was fired from six or eight jobs within the last year, someone who's been in [name of a mental health facility] ten times, okay, someone who's been in and out of the [mental] hospital, someone that's on five and six kinds of medications and would have to be coming back and forth to the hospital or the center here which would interfere with employment.

By teaching inexperienced informants what is and is not relevant information, protecting their identities, and referring to them respectfully, perhaps officially as "special employees" (but as "snitches" in private), detectives also maintain professional relations with their referral sources (Skolnick, 1966: 129-133).

By managing referrals, counselors not only created a supply of potential cases to work but also controlled (in some fashion) the kinds of cases to be worked. While counselors certainly worked with individuals whose disabilities were severe and whose likelihood of becoming employed was minimal (and admired those who wanted to work despite the odds), counselors typically did not seek to establish referral sources that provided such cases primarily.[5] Like other human service professionals, such as those of a community mental health center in a large eastern city who "warded off" "bad cases" by managing referral sources (Lang, 1981), rehabilitation counselors sought "good cases" to work. While many of the cases counselors worked were something other than "good," and some that seemed good later turned out not to be, counselors stressed the importance of good referrals and good referral sources. Referral sources were good when they provided a sufficient supply of good referrals, that is, individuals who wanted to work, could benefit from and realized the benefit of obviously needed services (which might be relatively inexpensive), and whose cases could be made and concluded relatively quickly (relative to the kinds of cases with which the counselors routinely worked). For example, the counselor who developed the military base as a referral source described the referrals from that source as "good" because records were readily available to demonstrate that the referrals possessed disabilities. Therefore, it was "merely a matter of finding out whether they [the referrals] could be potentially employable." In contrast were "walk-ins," who might not remember where they last worked and were uncertain as to what bothered them. It might take "months and months of trying to more or less fish around and figure out" if the applicants were eligible or not. Similarly, because of "bad referrals" from the Social Security Administration of "hostile," "angry" individuals whose disability benefits had been terminated, one counselor "had to get another referral source." By successfully managing referrals, counselors made managing their caseloads a less difficult task.

As one counselor who obtained many referrals yearly, many of which were "good" referrals, noted:

> Again, I'm fortunate that my referral sources—We have very good working relationships, and they provide me with whatever I need from them as far as places [to see referrals, applicants, and clients] and those type things. They are more than willing for me to come and set up my offices there and do what I want to do, which is very helpful.

ORGANIZING WORK

Detectives typically receive more cases from patrol than they can handle effectively. Therefore, they need to decide whether or not to investigate a case and, if so, how much. Through these decisions they begin to organize their work. Detectives use informal rules, such as the important case rule and the workable case rule, as guidelines for deciding which cases to work and, equally important, as justifications for why they are working certain cases (Sanders, 1977; Waegel, 1981). Rehabilitation counselors and other human service professionals also organize their work, though deciding which cases to work and which not to work is only part of those organizing efforts (see Chapter 3).

With often more than 100 cases pressing for attention, and with concerns that transcended any one of those cases, rehabilitation counselors organized their work. They did so be means of several interrelated strategies. Among them were *controlling their caseloads, catching up,* and *using priorities.*

Controlling the Caseload

Counselors wanted to be "on top" of their caseloads, to be aware of where their cases were within the rehabilitation process and to make sure their cases were progressing in a timely manner through that process. For example, had a general medical report been received yet? Had the applicant been vocationally evaluated yet? Was the case ready to be staffed for plan? How was the client's job search going? Was the case ready to be closed? These questions would be relatively easy to answer for an individual case. What made the task difficult, of course, was the fact that these questions needed to be answered for more than 100 and sometimes more than 200 cases. Counselors used two basic strategies in trying to control their caseloads: *reactive* and *proactive* control.

As noted earlier in this chapter, the distinction between reactive and proactive law enforcement concerns who initiates the enforcement activities. When reactive, law enforcement officers are responding to the actions of others who have asked for their assistance. Citizens complain and officers are dispatched to the scenes of the crimes, officers write field reports to which detectives respond. When proactive, law enforcement personnel combat crime through their own initiative. Through "speed traps," observation of suspects while patrolling, undercover work, and the like, law enforcement officials enforce the law proactively. While rehabilitation counselors tend to be much more proactive than detectives in obtaining cases to work, their stance changes somewhat when they manage their caseloads.

With typically more than 100 cases to manage at any time, many counselors found it difficult to remain current on all of them. Therefore, much of their control effort was reactive. As reports (such as a medical examination or a workshop evaluation) came to the counselor's attention or as applicants, clients, and other involved parties contacted the counselors, counselors responded (if possible) by doing whatever needed to be done (for example, staff the medical examination with the medical consultant) to move the case forward. In responding to "brush fires," as one counselor called the more significant, unplanned interruptions (such as the possibility of a client's electricity being cut off), counselors organized their work. Or, as one counselor noted metaphorically, "The screeching wheels will get the oil." However, what happened if the wheels did not screech (although the vehicle was not progressing smoothly)? There was danger in controlling a caseload reactively, a danger counselors did not always avoid: the *nonresponse*. Whether it was no response from an applicant/client or from someone else by whom the counselor expected to be contacted (such as a doctor who was to send a report of a medical examination), if no word was received on a case, then it might languish in the counselor's files. Cases might sit for months with no action taken because nothing had come across the counselors' desks to which they might respond. In an unusual case, a counselor admitted to a colleague that he had "forgotten" about a case in his file. When he happened to see the case, he tried to contact the client, was unable to do so, and thus closed the case as an unsuccessful closure. The counselor had not had any contact with the client for almost a year. Reactive rehabilitation put control of counselors' caseloads in the often uncertain and unsteady hands of the applicants, clients, and other involved parties.[6]

Consequently, counselors also tried to manage their caseloads proactively.[7] During the course of my research, I learned of several who were developing or learning techniques in order to be more proactive. As one counselor noted of a monitoring system she was being taught by a state office professional: "It really gives me a feeling of control as far as me being in control of the caseload, instead of the caseload controlling me." A counselor who typically worked with severely disabled clients would have advised new counselors to be an active person, not reactive to what's happening. You lose control when you become reactive. . . . You have to initiate the response, not let things come to you. That's when you get yourself in a lot of trouble, being inactive . . . just because a client is not on your case that doesn't mean you're not on his case.

In order to be on a "client's case," counselors needed to keep track of the progress of their cases. Counselors used different techniques in proactively controlling their caseloads, some of which were more systematic than others. Some counselors used a monitoring system developed by a professional in the state office, whereby the status of each case was reviewed periodically, what needed to be done next noted, and the subsequent review date indicated in a ledger. Some reviewed their cases with their casework assistants. Others "tried" to go through their caseloads periodically to stay on top of each case. One counselor attempted to go through all cases in referral status every month and those in active status (those for whom a plan had been written) every two to three months, because the counselor had about 30 of the former and 100 of the latter. And another counselor, during an interview in December, noted that he was going through his active cases to make certain there were no "sleepers" among them (cases in which contact had not been made since September).[8] However, the counselors were not always successful in getting through their caseloads, as I observed instances in which gaps in counselors' documentations were longer than the time limit they allowed themselves to review their cases.

When proactive control of their caseloads was successful, counselors not only felt in control of their caseloads but were also less likely to have gaps in their documentation, which also meant they were less likely to have gaps in their contact with their applicants and clients. Applicants and clients might also have been better aware of what was happening on their cases. According to one counselor, she was receiving fewer phone calls from applicants, who were now being informed of what was happening on their cases as the counselor reviewed them.

Catching Up

With all the cases counselors managed, it was not surprising that they sometimes fell behind. Vacations (before or after), twice-yearly audits (which could often be anticipated in advance), impending transfer to another caseload or another position within the agency, or anticipated departure from the agency were often reasons for counselors to get their caseloads in order.[9] Counselors tried to catch up on their work and on their documentation, which, as noted in the previous chapter, was partially a window to their otherwise invisible work. By entering previous contacts that had yet to be written, as well as by making contacts when recent ones had yet to be made, counselors organized their activities to present an orderly view of their work. One counselor sequestered himself once a month in another office and had his assistant handle calls and messages so that he could catch up on his work. In catching up, counselors tried to manage their caseloads better, but at times this procedure meant that clients were served less well. One counselor explained why audits were "devastating":

> The amount of time that people take away from clients to get ready for audits. I think that's the part that they don't understand, that nobody in rehabilitation is ever caught up, and so, if you hear of an audit coming, everything stops, and you start getting your R-1s up to snuff.

No doubt detectives who don't want their "red numbers" (numbers assigned to cases so that supervisors can monitor compliance with deadlines for reports) to become overdue also must catch up with their (paper)work (Waegel, 1981). Undoubtedly, so must caseworkers in the intake division of a public welfare agency who do not want their case investigations into applicants' entitlements and needs to become delinquent (Zimmerman, 1966: chap. 6; however, see Prottas, 1979: 41-42).

Priorities

Typically faced with many cases to handle and a great deal to do (though it is not always done), human service professionals establish priorities in deciding which cases to handle and what to do (Emerson and Pollner, 1978; Peyrot, 1982). For example, psychiatric emergency teams (PET) in a community health clinic in Southern California selected emergencies on file to investigate according to their sense of what was most serious, urgent, or the "worst." Yet this priority was often "subordinated to and/or completely dismissed in favor of a ranking reflecting a variety of organizational and personal needs and prin-ciples," such as "any case [would] do" when the PET professionals were "pressed to meet a weekly production quota or when facing admin-istrative criticism for allowing a backlog of cases to accumulate" (Emerson and Pollner, 1978: 91, 98).

As noted earlier in this section, detectives use guidelines, such as the important case rule and the workable case rule, in setting priorities. When detectives are working "hot" cases (good cases with leads), they may give relatively little attention to new cases they receive (Sanders 1977: 136). Rehabilitation counselors also used priorities in allocating their time and efforts, priorities that developed out of organizational concerns.

While the counselors' priorities varied somewhat (and may be put aside in the face of "brush fires," impending audits, and other contingencies), counselors often stressed "production" activities: job placement (such as providing tools for a client whose employment was soon to begin), plans (developing them and serving the clients), and successful closures (monitoring and preparing to close cases). As one counselor remarked, she and her colleagues got "brownie points for putting people to work." They also got those "brownie points" for plans (which preceded the placement) and closures (which followed the placement). "Production" activities did not necessarily mean paper-work, though paperwork was needed to move applicants/clients officially into various statuses. Critical rehabilitation activities such as job placement, vocational evaluation, development of a plan of services, and job follow-up were involved in "production." As one counselor noted, "When you're dealing with people, you have to do what needs to be done with people; paperwork can wait." It generally did, except to the extent that it was necessary for production activities.

In organizing their work according to priorities, counselors might keep a list of potential closures, circle calendar dates when cases could be closed, or separate the folders of those who were working from the other folders (and place the former in open view) so that these important cases would not be forgotten. At the beginning of each month, some counselors planned which cases they would be able to close or put into plan status during the month. Some tried to do plans and closures at the beginning of the month (though "any system you make is open to barrage from every corner," according to one counselor), and one counselor could "go through the month much easier" if she accomplished those plans and closures (approximately one-twelfth of the yearly goals) at the beginning. These production concerns typically would be attended to before routine paperwork (such as catching up on R-1 notes), closing cases status 08 or 28 (see Prottas, 1979: 41-42, for similar priorities of intake workers in a public welfare agency), trying to track a client who had not been in contact with the agency for months or even years (which gets "bottom priority," according to one counselor), and other tasks. For example:

While discussing an IWRP with an applicant, a counselor learned that the applicant would begin work in five days. The counselor told the applicant that he would try to "rush" to get the plan approved in order to provide her work clothes in time for her to begin work. After the client left, the counselor completed the evaluation summary of the IWRP and then asked his casework assistant to give this plan "priority" so that it could be approved by the local and state QC in time to provide the work clothes to the client when she needed them.

The counselors' priorities became particularly apparent and important as the end of the fiscal year approached. Counselors who were behind in their goals, particularly closures, began to organize their efforts toward "getting their goals." Counselors emphasized getting clients into status 22, employed, because clients needed to work a minimum of sixty days before their cases could be closed. Counselors went through their caseloads to make sure all potential 26s were closed as such. One counselor made a special visit to a small town he did not regularly go to in order to get some closures. As the end of the fiscal year approached, counselors were urged to "get their closures in," even if that meant neglecting some of their other activities. Transferred cases, referrals, and even plans, if counselors were heavily pressed, might be put on hold as counselors directed their efforts to "getting their [closure] goals." Several counselors declined to allow me to accompany them because they were too busy with the approaching end of the fiscal year. One counselor described at the beginning of May what it would be like until the end of the fiscal year, June 30:

> I will be working on Saturdays until July 1. Then I am going to take the summer off. Really . . . there is a lot you have to do. I don't know why it always seems to fall the very last part of the fiscal year because we do it ourselves. . . . I worked real hard this spring [on] placements, so there will be cases to close this last two months. Sorta worked the first few months on getting people . . . evaluated, in plan, and ready for placement, and then it kinda got to that stage in February, March, and April, and now a lot of them are working. So I am going to have make sure my documentation is up to date on them and, you know, keep checking with them and make sure that everything is going okay and then finally do the closure on them.

As another counselor explained, in looking back at the end of the fiscal year:

> I have really spent most of this month [June] trying to meet production for this year. As you know, the end of the fiscal year we're having to take a

review and see what we can do, where we are with our goals for the year. And we were expected to close [number] cases this year. We were short of that at the beginning of the month, and so we had to work very—we had to put that as top priority for the month. We had to let everything else go and concentrate totally on meeting that goal. And that was quite a job to do, but we did it, we finished that last week. We did meet our goal. So right now I'm trying to sit back and take a look at where I've got to go. I've got just a tremendous amount of paperwork to do. I've got about 25 plans now that I can write, IWRPs that I can write, that we've evaluated, they're eligible, and we need to go ahead and write those up and get things going there.

This emphasis on producing closures to meet goals as the end of the fiscal year approached was reflected clearly in the cumulative percentage of cases closed each month during the fiscal year. If successful closures were achieved evenly throughout the fiscal year, then approximately one-twelfth (or 8.33 percent) of the total closures for the year would be achieved each month. This is not what happened. While percentages varied from counselor to counselor, both officewide and statewide proportionately more cases were closed successfully in the last three months of the fiscal year, particularly in the last month, than earlier in the year. Plans, however, were written at a more even pace throughout the fiscal year. Table 5.1 provides the expected (based on an even production of plans and closures) and observed cumulative percentages for the production of plans and successful closures for a recent year in the area office I studied. The pattern for this year is even less dramatic than those for other fiscal years of the late 1970s and early 1980s that I was able to calculate. In one recent year almost 25 percent of the total number of successful cases closed were closed in the *last* month of the fiscal year.

Table 5.1 suggests an important effect of counselors' emphasis on getting closures at the end of the fiscal year. That emphasis was likely to be *self-perpetuating*. With so much effort placed on closing cases and with the possible neglect of other activities (such as obtaining referrals, evaluating referrals, and so on), counselors were likely to have relatively few cases to close at the beginning of the new fiscal year. They began the fiscal year "behind" and spent the rest of it trying to catch up. In catching up at the end of the fiscal year, they depleted their caseloads of clients whose cases could have been closed as successfully rehabilitated early in the next fiscal year, and they allowed other kinds of casework that needed to be attended to before cases could be made or concluded successfully in the new fiscal year to pile up. Some counselors attributed this "catch-up" to not yet having enough time (about three or four years) to develop the caseload properly (that is, to have an adequate flow of

TABLE 5.1
Cumulative Percentage of Observed and Expected Production
of Plans and Successful Closures

| | Observed | | Expected |
	Plans	Closures	
July	8	4	8
August	17	10	17
September	22	15	25
October	33	27	33
November	41	33	42
December	47	40	50
January	56	51	58
February	62	57	67
March	71	65	75
April	82	76	83
May	90	86	92
June	100	100	100

referrals and an even pace of rehabilitation activities), though at least one counselor, who was transferred to several different caseloads during my research, managed to "turn around" some poorly producing caseloads within one fiscal year.[10]

Certainly not all counselors were caught up in this fiscal-year cycle of "catch-up." Some successful counselors had reversed the cycle. They closed a relatively large proportion of successful cases in the first part of the fiscal year, met their goals well before the end of the fiscal year (by weeks, a month, even more), and then prepared for the next fiscal year by lining up plans and closures for the next fiscal year.[11] For some counselors, getting a head start on the upcoming fiscal year was a luxury they had only recently begun to enjoy. And one counselor who would not quite meet his closure goals for the present fiscal year was looking forward to the next because he had some closures "in the kitty" (cases soon to be closed successfully). Whether counselors made closures in the early parts of the fiscal year or rushed at the end, the priority of production was used in organizing their work.

PACE OF THE CASE(LOAD)

Detectives work cases that vary greatly in how quickly they are disposed of. Some cases are inactivated after a few contacts. The victim is contacted and a follow-up report written that inactivates the case due to a lack of investigative leads. Other cases, such as "whodunits" in which the detectives have no initial idea of who killed the victim, may be investigated for months or even kept open for years (Sanders, 1977: 173-174). The pace of the case varies not only from case to case but also more generally from one detective detail to another. Detectives who work major crimes, such as homicides, robberies, and rapes, might "work for days, weeks, or months on the same case even if there is only a slim chance it will be solved" (Sanders, 1977: 168). However, detectives who handle juvenile offenses or work the burglary detail might dispose of a case (inactivate it due to no investigative leads) after a contact or two.

The pace of cases and caseloads was also important to the rehabilitation counselors I observed. Some cases were made and concluded quickly, in a few months; others took many months, even many years, to be made and concluded. For example, when the agency was (heavily) involved in "bill paying," many cases moved relatively rapidly: the applicants were working, surgery or medical services were provided, and then the clients resumed their jobs. They were "quick-turnover" cases. While those "bill-paying" cases became much less frequent, counselors still handled cases that turned over relatively quickly. Cooperative adult applicants who wanted to get back to work or who were working, but whose jobs were in jeopardy because of their disabilities, whose medical information was obtained easily and whose services would not be protracted (such as counseling and guidance with some medical follow-up) might be quick-turnover cases. Of course, unforeseen disruptions could and did occur. Students, applicants who were severely disabled, those with little work history, and those to be trained would be longer-term cases.

Just as the pace of cases varied from one detective detail to another, so did the pace vary among rehabilitation counselors' caseloads. School caseloads and particularly the specialty caseload of disability benefit recipients were slower paced. School-aged clients might be served for several years as they moved through high school before they were placed on a job. Some, of course, enrolled in postsecondary educational institutions, which prolonged their cases. Cases that involved recipients of disability benefits from the Social Security Administration (SSDI and SSI recipients) were particularly slow moving. Applicants might be evaluated for months, as long as eighteen months in extended evaluation, before a plan was even developed. They might then be served for years before their cases were closed. As one counselor who handled such a caseload explained:

I like working with this caseload because it's real slow paced. It's not a high-turnover. You get to know your clients well. Like on a general caseload, you don't get to know your clients well because it's very fast paced. The client might come in today, and the case might be closed three months later or four months later. I work some of these people for years.

A slower-paced, low-turnover caseload would also have lower goals to meet.

In great contrast to slower-paced caseloads were the caseloads, whether officially designated as specialty or not, that consisted of public offenders. This specialty caseload is discussed in greater detail in the next chapter. Here, its relatively rapid pace will be mentioned briefly. Public offender caseloads did a "high-volume" business. Because the cases turned over relatively quickly, they had the highest goals in the state. The field counselor typically received such cases in plan status, the plans having been developed by rehabilitation counselors who worked inside correctional facilities. Much of the guidance and counseling provided on the cases had been provided in correctional facilities as well. After the offenders were released, some were never seen again. Others, however, obtained employment, were issued a second maintenance check (the first having been issued when they were released) and perhaps some work clothes and tools, and were contacted once or twice on their jobs before their cases were closed. Field counselors were involved primarily in concluding the cases, not in making them.

Ironically, some of the counselors who managed caseloads consisting of disability benefit recipients were assigned to public offender caseloads during the course of my research. The difference in pace was striking to them and not completely welcomed. One such counselor, who recently had been assigned public offenders, explained the contrast:

You might talk to them [clients receiving disability benefits] today and not talk to them . . . till two months later and nothing really has changed that much. But with these people [the ex-offenders], you have to . . . pretty much stay on your toes with them . . . or you're just going to lose contact with them.

Contact often was lost, as I discuss in the next chapter.

Moving Cases Quickly

While the pace of cases and caseloads varied, counselors typically attempted to move cases quickly through the rehabilitation process.

They did so for both making and concluding cases, particularly perhaps for the former. While critics have argued that processing cases quickly is caused by the emphasis on production (see Chapter 1), that criticism is an oversimplification. No doubt some counselors, giving little thought to the clients, did sometimes work cases quickly to "get their goals." For example, a counselor who worked in another area office was criticized for rushing applicants into plan status and then "picking up" additional disabilities and problems as they were uncovered rather than thoroughly evaluating the applicants before developing a plan. I observed cases in which supervisory personnel and consultants required counselors to evaluate applicants further before developing a plan. These latter observations point both to the orientation to move cases quickly and to the agency's (and the counselors') concern that to do so too quickly would not serve the interests of the disabled individuals. Counselors themselves complained that applicants, not realizing the system through which counselors had to work, expected the process to go more quickly than was possible. Some expected services or jobs immediately and were often disappointed if the process moved slowly. It was this issue, and not solely the concern with production, that was the basis for the counselors' concern in moving cases quickly.

Clients and closures could be lost through delay. If applicants who came looking for help (sometimes after finding no help elsewhere, or after making a personally difficult decision to seek help) were asked to wait too long as medical records and evaluations were sought, openings developed for evaluation at the rehabilitation center, appointments scheduled, and services finally rendered, then their initial motivation, enthusiasm, and commitment might wane as the delay grew. Infrequently, they might find jobs on their own. Neither counselors nor supervisory personnel wanted cases languishing in status "02," application made, or in statuses "10" and "12," the plan written but not yet implemented.[12] Therefore, though they were not always successful, counselors often attempted to move cases promptly (to provide services in a "timely" manner, as the agency put it).[13]

One counselor explained how he worked cases:

As quickly as the information comes in, I don't hold things at all. If I get the report today, then I staff it today. If not, I might wait till next . . . day [the day when the counselor's staffing group met] depending again on how urgent things seem. There are no cases that have been ready for plan for a couple of months that are just still . . . sitting there. That just never happens.

And, as the counselor added,

One thing I think about is: How can I make it possible for us to get what needs to be done face to face in as few sessions as possible?

Counselors might move cases quickly in a variety of ways.[14] They might use various strategies to obtain quickly needed medical information. Instead of beginning with a general medical evaluation, one counselor authorized an internist's exam if it was "clear" the referral's problem was "high blood pressure." Doing so would provide the needed information and save time and money (that is, a general medical evaluation and the specialist's examination would not be used, only the latter). Counselors who routinely worked a federal hospital as a referral source became unpaid consultants so they could photocopy the medical records (and other pertinent information) of their applicants. This often enabled them to staff for plan cases they had opened only a few days previously. In order to move a case quickly, one counselor put an applicant on the waiting list for an evaluation at the rehabilitation center even though the applicant was at that time heavily medicated due to a psychological disability. The counselor who did this planned to follow the applicant closely until the time of the applicant's entrance into the workshop. The counselor believed this was preferable to not getting an entry date until the applicant was "ready" to be evaluated, which would then mean several more months of waiting to enter the facility. Instead of waiting for openings at the workshop, other counselors might do their own evaluations with paper-and-pencil tests and counseling sessions. Moving cases quickly might even involve the advice of one counselor to another to contact, in person, a doctor who had failed to send the report of a visual examination of an applicant, or to cancel the authorization for the examination and not mention the visual impairment of the applicant when staffing the case for the plan *because* the impairment did not pose a vocational handicap. If the applicant was leaving a treatment facility that served as a referral source, then the counselor might open a case and develop a plan with the applicant on the same day. Or, if counselors needed to provide some service "yesterday," then, instead of waiting for their next regularly scheduled case development staffing, they might staff a case with their QC or several colleagues.

Supervisory personnel were equally concerned with the potential problems of delays in evaluating and serving applicants and clients. For example, during the course of my research, the local area office established a procedure designed to speed up the psychological evaluation of applicants. Instead of necessarily setting up appointments for their applicants to be seen personally by the staff psychologist, counselors could staff the applicants' cases with the psychologist to establish a disability and to develop a program of services. With sufficient information in the applicants' folders (such as IQ test results and school reports), the psychologist could enable the counselors to make a case that bypassed probable missed appointments, saved several weeks in the process, and probably saved many cases that would not have been made because of the applicants' reluctance to see a psychologist. However, as one professional involved noted, under the new procedures the psychologist became familiar with the applicant's folder, not necessarily with the applicant.

Once cases were made, counselors remained concerned about serving clients in a timely manner. Again, delays could mean disaster. Counselors might begin to provide guidance and counseling to clients before the IWRP had been approved by the state office. Authorizations for work clothes, tools, and other needed items were often processed with the priority of serving clients in a timely manner. "Brush fires" were put out as counselors became aware of them. In attempting to handle one brush fire, a counselor and I staked out a client's apartment:

> While in the field on a job follow-up visit, a counselor who worked with hearing—impaired individuals called her casework assitant and learned that a company that had decided to hire one of her clients that morning wanted the client to undergo a routine physical examination in two hours. The counselor would have to pick up her client, take him to the company within an hour and a half to obtain some forms and then to the examination at four o'clock. We drove to the client's residence, knocked on what we thought was the client's door, but were told by a woman who answered that no such person lived there. Instead, the woman pointed us "up the street." The woman was mistaken. We came back, knocked on the other door of the duplex, but no one answered. We went back to the woman and asked if she knew where the *deaf* individual lived. "Next door," she said. Either the client had not heard us or was not at home. The counselor called a colleague at the rehabilitation center who brought with him the roommate of the counselor's client, who happened to be a client himself. The roommate went into the apartment, but the client was not there, and the roommate did not know where he would be. The counselor, the counselor's colleague, and I circled the neighborhood, but we did not see the client. The colleague returned to the workshop, but the counselor and I remained for another 45 minutes in her car across the street from the client's home. The client did not show, but later that afternoon alternative arrangements were made for the client to "take the physical" and begin work the following week.

Through their own strategies, other human service professionals, such as intake workers in a public welfare agency, move cases quickly too

(Zimmerman, 1966: 210). So do detectives when handling routine cases and trying both to meet deadlines for submitting investigative reports and to produce arrests (Waegel, 1981).

"Delaying" Cases

While counselors attempted to move cases quickly, sometimes they deliberately slowed the pace of the case. They "walked" rather than "ran," to use one counselor's phrase. When counselors had misgivings about an applicant's or client's commitment to rehabilitation, they moved the case more slowly. For example, if applicants had been drinking, some counselors would not see them. Not only might the "alcohol be talking instead of the applicants," but had the applicants "really" made a commitment to addressing their problems? Or, evaluations could be used to check whether or not applicants were "sincere":

At one case development staffing a counselor asked for suggestions about the following case: an applicant who had been on a wide variety of drugs for more than ten years was now in a local treatment facility where he would be for approximately four months. According to the counselor, the applicant was trying to "clean up his act." Another counselor wondered if the applicant had actually reformed. "Only time would tell." Therefore, why not send the applicant to the rehabilitation facility where, during the applicant's evaluation, his reformation could be checked.

Additional evaluations and adjustment services were also used to check on and better prepare clients who were doing poorly in finding and/or maintaining employment. When counselors suspected that applicants or clients were using the agency to obtain tangibles without having made a commitment to rehabilitate themselves, counselors might delay paperwork or double-check the applicant's or client's story before arranging for those tangibles. For example, when they suspected the client would "take the money and run," counselors might delay providing a maintenance check. Other counselors might "sit" on the case of a "hostile and demanding" client who had not gotten along with four previous counselors. Counselors "ran" and "walked" in trying to manage their caseloads successfully. No doubt, when detectives and other human service professionals work "sensitive" cases or become skeptical about the case and those involved, they too "walk" rather than "run."

THE STAFFING

While detectives often work cases on their own, they do assist each other in important ways. Many detectives and other law enforcement officers do, of course, work the same major crime. More routinely, detectives share information within and across details. For example, narcotics detectives who, looking for drugs, have "raided" a dwelling might inform burglary detectives that they observed many television sets or other often-burglarized items. Or one detectives might fill in another detective who was working a case that involved a complainant or suspect with whom the first detective was familiar. Detectives may even staff cases. When they assemble in the morning they are likely to read the morning's batch of patrol reports, "commenting on them, trying to decide which ones should be worked and which ones shouldn't" (Sanders, 1977: 77). Or, after investigators of a West Coast-city Sex Crime Unit arrived each morning, "they would go together with the sergeant for a coffee break where they would discuss cases and where the sergeant would sometimes ask who was available to take new cases" (Sanders, 1980: 87). Perhaps more so than for detectives, the staffing is an integral and important feature of the work of rehabilitation counselors and other human service professionals (Buckholdt and Gubrium, 1979a, 1979b).

Counselors routinely staffed cases with the medical consultant and staff psychologist, with the staff of the rehabilitation center (for evaluation and services), and with their fellow counselors in case development staffings. Counselors' dealings with the medical consultant and staff psychologist and their use of the rehabilitation center have been noted earlier. The case development staffing, also known as the CDS, concerns me here.

Through the CDS (and other staffings), the agency intended that professionals (sometimes from different disciplines) would "share their knowledge and expertise to arrive at a unified plan of action." Case development staffings were held weekly and were scheduled for one-hour periods. Groups consisting of approximately five to seven counselors (composition of the groups changed throughout my research) met, were led by a quality control specialist or the area supervisor, and were assisted (routinely in the new office, irregularly in the former area office, whose staff and counselors were greatly reduced in numbers) by a casework assistant who recorded in the R-1 notes the course of action that had been agreed upon. Counselors were required to staff cases they intended to close 08 or 28 or those they intended to put into plan.[15] Cases about which counselors were uncertain could also be staffed "for direction." Cases to be closed as successfully rehabilitated, status 26, did not need to be staffed. Unless they were unsure about the status, counselors rarely staffed such cases. As one counselor remarked to me, "You don't get to see the successes in the CDS." No, but what you did get to see was one aspect of their work necessary for successes as well as inside talk about other aspects of their work.

While 08s, 28s, and plans had to be staffed in CDS, concurrence was only a necessary, not a sufficient, condition for final agency approval. The local QC would review all three kinds of cases before referring them to the state office, where additional QCs would review the third kind before they were approved. As QCs told counselors on various occasions, particularly in reference to plans, they would have a chance to check them again when the cases came across their desks. What seemed acceptable when presented orally in CDS might look different on paper. Information that might have caused the QC to question the intended course of action (such as an alternative vocational objective incompatible with the applicant's disability) might not have been mentioned or its significance not fully realized. As one QC said of the counselors:

> They have an idea of what they want to do, and some of them are very experienced. I'm not saying they are trying to pull the wool over us, but . . . there's a lot you can say. So I say a lot of times, "Based on what you tell me, you know, this sounds like what we need to do . . ."

While counselors staffed cases somewhat differently depending on the intended course of action (plan or closure) and their certainty about that action and themselves, their staffings followed a general pattern. The counselor often introduced the case by providing some brief information about the case, such as the applicant's/client's age, sex, perhaps race, sometimes name, referral source, and disability. The information was provided so others present would have some understanding of the case and could comment on it. If the counselor had not prefaced this background information with the intended course of action (such as "I'd like to 08 this case"), then the counselor would state the intended course of action and justify it. When staffing plans, some counselors read from their already-written plans, while others, as they flipped through the case folders, related the facts of the cases and what they intended to do. Counselors infrequently staffed cases in a batch. Cases that were similar in the important features relating to the intended course of action might be staffed as a batch. If not staffed as a batch, the counselor might comment on the similarity of some cases or on the fact that one case was similar to a previous one. For example, cases to be closed 08 in which the counselor had made a personal contact to determine if the applicants were interested in services, but had found the applicants were not, might be staffed as a batch. Or a counselor might staff as a batch several cases that were to be put into plan and that were very similar, such as cases in which the applicants had psychological disabilities but no physical problems, medical information had been secured, and counseling and guidance and job placement would be provided.

Counselors also infrequently "contingency staffed" their cases. If a particular event occurred, then the counselor planned to handle the case a certain way. Closures in 08 and 28 status were sometimes contingency staffed: The cases would be closed contingent upon an additional attempt to contact the applicants or clients. Even a plan might be contingency staffed. For example, a counselor intended to develop a plan contingent upon the medical consultant's assessment that an applicant with residuals of cancer (such as shortness of breath, cardiac arrhythmia, and chest pains) did have functional limitations that constituted a vocational handicap. However, supervisory personnel often did not favor such contingency staffing. Instead, counselors were urged to have "all" their information before they staffed a case, especially if the information was "crucial" and potentially problematic, as in the contingent plan described above.

Justifying Intentions

When staffing cases, counselors justified their intended courses of action. Doing so seems to be a necessary, routine feature of human service work where accountability is so accentuated (Gubrium and Buckholdt, 1982: chap 6). Without adequate justification (that is, adequate in the opinion of those who passed judgment, such as the QC), counselors could not proceed upon the intended course of action. Counselors might provide matter-of-fact, obvious-to-all justifications. For example, as a justification for an 08 closure, one counselor stated, "This guy is gainfully employed and doesn't want our services." Other justifications might be equally matter-of-factly provided and accepted, though not nearly so brief.

In other cases, the intended course of action and (by implication, though also explicitly) the justifications were questioned by members of the CDS, particularly the QC or the area supervisor. Extended discussions might follow in which the counselor in charge of the case, sometimes with the assistance of colleagues, would try to rejustify the intended course of action. Sometimes these additional justifications were accepted. For example, a counselor, noting that the client had previously worked as a cashier at a department store,

> staffed a case for a plan with the vocational objectives of cashier and office worker. The QC wondered what the counselor had to "back up" office worker as an objective. The counselor noted that when the client began working at the department store she began with the billing system and then switched to cashier. Another counselor suggested that the applicant be tested to make sure that her reading competence and interest matched the objectives. The QC wondered, however, how long the applicant had worked as a cashier. Told that it had been seven years, the QC concluded that additional testing was not needed.

At other times the counselor was required to "do more" (for example, to obtain another evaluation or make another attempt to contact the applicant) before pursuing the originally intended course of action. And at still other times the intended course of action might be changed dramatically. What a counselor intended as an 08 might be recast as a possible plan, a plan recast perhaps as an 08, though certainly needing more investigation if it were to be a plan, and a 28 recast as a possible 26, a successful closure, as the following case illustrates:

> A counselor staffed a case for 28 closure. The client had been provided counseling and guidance toward a vocational objective of cashier. The client's husband had died in an automobile accident. When in the counselor's office, she cried uncontrollably. Through "C and G" she no longer did so. However, the client met a man, lived with that man, and took care of the man's son and her own daughter. The client was not returning to work. Another counselor suggested that a successful closure as a homemaker might be appropriate. The QC noted that if the counselor felt that she had provided services which enabled the client to perform her homemaking duties well, then a 26 closure would be appropriate. A third counselor urged the counselor in charge to see the case as follows: The client came to you, the counselor, when the client was in need, you helped her, and now she has entered into a meaningful relation with another person and is taking care of children. Therefore, you have provided a service. The QC noted that the counselor in charge was the only one who knew if the 26 closure would be legitimate or not. Therefore, the counselor should take another look at her case.

Cases mentioned in the previous two chapters also illustrate how they could be recast through discussion. Both the acceptance and rejection of justifications addressed the acceptable ways of working and concluding cases (see the previous two chapters).

Because justifications were important, questions might arise when counselors (or casework assistants) staffed cases for colleagues who were not present. Documentation in the case folders, particularly the R-1 notes, might not have adequately explained and justified the counselors' intended courses of action (see Chapter 4). Without personal knowledge of the case, the substitute counselor (and to a lesser extent the CWA, who would be partly familiar with the case) would have difficulty filling in the gaps in the paper reasoning. In these instances the cases might have to be restaffed by the absent counselors or they might be asked to support more fully their intended courses of action by providing additional explanation. For example, at one staffing,

> a counselor staffed a case for an absent colleague who intended to put the case into plan with vocational objectives of janitor and laborer. The documentation in the folder indicated that the applicant had previously worked as a laborer but wanted to change vocations. The QC wondered why "janitor" had been listed as the primary objective. While the client could "probably handle" that job according to the QC, the QC asked the counselor who was staffing the case to write a note to the counselor in charge asking that the latter document in his R-1 notes "how he arrived at janitor."

Because justifications concerning, discussions of, and explanations about cases varied greatly, so did the lengths of time devoted to the cases. Some cases were presented in less than a minute, some in only a few seconds, with no discussion by others. The lengthiest discussion I observed, 20 minutes long, concerned the case mentioned in Chapter 3 in which the client had not been provided all the scheduled psychotherapy sessions, but the CDS debated whether a 28 or a 26 closure was appropriate. At the next week's CDS, the counselor in charge of the case mentioned that, after additional contact with the client, she was satisfied with a 26. However, while there was great variation among cases, overall they were staffed quickly. Discussion lasted less than 3 minutes per case.[16] One QC noted that if counselors knew their cases and had the information organized, then it was not difficult to staff cases quickly. However, even in 3 minutes an important discussion can take place, as defendants and other concerned parties know from their criminal court experiences (President's Commission, 1967: 7; Gilsinan, 1982: 175).

Using the Staffing[17]

Counselors used the case development staffings for two major purposes: to *conduct the official business* of the agency and as a *social occasion* that expressed and supported the work of the counselors (and the agency). In staffings, counselors met formal requirements, staffed cases "for directions," obtained independent corroboration of their intended actions, and supported fellow counselors in their intended courses of action. By telling jokes and stories, counselors helped develop and maintain a shared identity and common bond.

As noted earlier, cases to be closed 08 or 28 or to be put into plan were required by the agency to be staffed. Thus counselors used staffings to meet the formal requirements of the agency. Cases that received little or no discussion (and were anticipated by counselors to be clear-cut) were staffed only because it was required. When they staffed cases, some counselors rarely received much feedback from their colleagues. And some experienced counselors felt that staffings were useful primarily for new counselors but not for them (unless they had a difficult case, and even then they could get advice from their colleagues). One such counselor felt that the staffing was a formality. He rarely asked for advice because he did not need it, and because the advice offered, if taken, would often slow the flow of the case. Once services were under way, an amendment to a plan could always be made later. Other counselors, not sure how to handle a case, would ask "for directions," for suggestions from their colleagues. Of course, unsolicited, but gratefully received, suggestions about how to manage cases were often provided by colleagues as well. Counselors also staffed cases to obtain independent corroboration for their intended courses of action, either explicitly to present to a doubting applicant or client, or simply to have available in case objections were later raised. In staffing for 08 closure (no vocational handicap) an applicant who had suffered a back injury and could not return to his original job but had improved greatly and was driving a taxi full time, a counselor remarked:

> He's balking a little bit. He's not being nasty about it, but he really is trying hard to understand why he's not eligible.... I told him I would staff it to make sure that I wasn't misinterpreting somewhere along the line.

And later:

> I told him I want to staff it for you so that I'm not sitting here and just me telling you this. I said I've got a good bit of training and a good bit of

experience behind me . . . so I am telling you what I feel is accurate, but I want to staff it for your own benefit.

And later:

I just don't think he is eligible for us. I want[ed] to find out if I was really crazy.

When counselors were not sure what to do, or when their intended courses of action were questioned by the QC or area supervisor, colleagues often supported their fellow counselors. They provided additional reasons for justifying an intended course of action, or they provided reasons for recasting 08s as plans or unsuccessful closures as successful ones. Though at times counselors certainly questioned their colleagues' intended courses of action, they often seemed to be supportive, even in their questioning. Sharing similar concerns and facing similar problems, counselors assisted one another in managing cases in the CDS. Cases mentioned in the previous chapters give testimony to that supportive colleagueship.

Finally, staffings were also a social occasion, where that colleagueship was reinforced. In sharing their work with one another and often its difficulties, counselors helped establish and maintain a shared identity and common bond. In the course of the staffings counselors gave *humorous expression to the demands and difficulties of their work*. One counselor told me that counselors needed to have a sense of humor and they did. They joked about putting into status 24 (services interrupted) a client who was sentenced to 40 years in prison. They joked that if there were a *Dictionary of Occupational Titles* code for "in jail," then, with that as a vocational objective, perhaps they could meet their goals. They kidded one another about "letting" applicants who were working become 08s instead of making cases (developing plans) on them. They kidded about traveling "to the beach" or out of state to track a client. One counselor joked about testing an applicant in a "wind tunnel" in order to make the applicant eligible. Another joked that before the CDSs took their present form, they used to staff ten cases at a time—08s, of course. One counselor facetiously remarked that a student applicant who had an IQ score of 74 was almost college material. That was not a "slam" against the student or colleges, but an indication that most of the applicants/clients with whom the counselor worked were much more severely retarded. Or, when a counselor wondered what reason should be used for closing an applicant's case 08, an applicant who wanted the agency to sponsor her graduate training (possibly out of state) but was not satisfied with "only" guidance and counseling for her emotional problems, a colleague kidded me, "Failure of VR to cooperate," a reversal of how counselors often closed applicants' cases. The joking and kidding did not serve to undermine the counselors' work, but to convey openly in a humorous, "safe," and yet also partly serious way their everyday concerns. Instead of "glossing" over those concerns, counselors acknowledged them humorously (Buckholdt and Gubrium, 1979b: 257).

Counselors also entertained their colleagues by recounting what an applicant or client had done or by reading from case materials. For example, in one staffing a counselor remarked:

> Okay, this is another of my famous 28s. This guy is a cell mate of the other guy I was just talking about. Let me tell you what this guy did. He was at [a juvenile training facility] and then he got released from [the training facility]. . . . He went down to [name] Church . . . and stole a silver chalice or something. Then he got sent up and did some time for that. He got parole. The week after he got parole he went back and stole the same thing. [Another counselor adds, "He's a glutton for punishment."] He's down there in [the county jail], and I think he's going to be there a while. They don't have any VR services down there.

Staffings were serious business, though those involved, whether rehabilitation counselors or other human service professionals, were not always serious in the staffings (Buckholdt and Gubrium, 1979a: chap. 5, 1979b).

However, detectives are not always serious when discussing crime, a generally serious topic. In one West Coast law enforcement department, the detectives sat around together reading the morning's batch of patrol reports:

> If a case involved someone who had been in habitual trouble, the detectives would comment on it, letting everyone know that so-and-so was at it again. If the case involved particularly funny circumstances, it would be read aloud for everyone's amusement [Sanders, 1977: 77].

Even detectives, involved in the most serious concerns, are not always serious. And sometimes serious concerns are expressed humorously, and, through that expression, support is provided for those concerns.

CONCLUSION

Detectives and other human service professionals work not only individual cases but handle many, sometimes hundreds of cases. They

5

MANAGING CASELOADS

During the course of a day, detective work "consists of a mosaic of little tasks," such as reading reports, looking for suspects, establishing crimes, going to court, catching up on paperwork, and making contacts (Sanders, 1977: 128). Each day, detectives may be handling many cases. While concluding the investigation on some, they are likely to receive new reports on others. They manage a mix of cases that they have worked to various stages in the investigative process. For example, in one sheriff's department on the West Coast, a detective in the juvenile detail handled more than 100 cases in a 12-week period, though many received "minimal investigative attention" (Sanders 1977: 133-134). Therefore, to understand detective work, one must understand not only how detectives work individual cases and conduct specific investigations, but also how they organize their efforts in dealing with many cases. This is particularly important for rehabilitation counselors and other human service professionals.

Rehabilitation counselors, like other human service professionals, have responsibility for many cases at the same time (Zimmerman, 1966: 257-261). In the course of a day, counselors may see several referrals, develop an IWRP, counsel a client, review medical records, and talk with an employer. They handle a mix of cases that are at different stages in the rehabilitation process and that may require different responses. In the office I investigated, rehabilitation counselors routinely managed more than 100 cases at a time, and more than 200 in the recent past. Counselors did not just work and conclude individual cases, they handled many cases simultaneously; they managed caseloads.

Counselors' concerns in managing their caseloads transcended the management of individual cases. They were assigned responsibility for

4. A GAO (1978: ii) audit of "third-party" funding agreements between state vocational rehabilitation agencies and other agencies serving disabled individuals, such as schools and hospitals, criticized such arrangements in part because the counselors "could lose control over the selection of clients to be served and the services provided." Accepting "bad" clients is not necessarily an indication of losing control, but rather is a means of developing control, a control based on mutual service. Another GAO (1982: 9-10) audit concluded that due to the influence (sometimes threats) of other programs, such as mental health facilities, counselors were accepting clients with little likelihood of benefiting from rehabilitation services in terms of employment. When counselors in the area office I observed accepted "bad" cases, it was not in response to a threat. Certainly, due to "political connections" and other special considerations, counselors sometimes worked with people they otherwise might not have. The GAO's criticism perhaps applies better to pretrial diversion programs in Boston, where, "dependent upon judges for referral and, indeed for their programs' existence, administrators found it difficult to refuse judges who referred too many clients, or inappropriate clients, to them" (Lipsky, 1980: 20).

5. One counselor who developed a referral source that primarily provided "bad" cases (cases, as seen by others, in which the individuals did not have a "reasonable" expectation of benefiting from the agency's service due to the severity of their disabilities) was criticized at times for poorly screening such cases. When the counselor left the agency, the succeeding counselor did not work that referral source very regularly.

6. In one parole agency, most parolees on the parole officers' caseloads were "paper men," men who had been judged by the POs as insincere but controllable, and those who had not been judged. POs saw their paper men only one or two times each year. One wonders how well these parolees were "controlled" (or served), especially if the POs mistakenly judged the men. A great deal of "control" must have been reactive, though the investigator does not say (McCleary, 1978: 126-127).

7. QCs tried to help them in doing so. Time and status reports, which informed counselors of how long each case was in its present status, could be used as a "very good tool" to control a caseload according to one QC. The QCs would make comments on counselors' time and status reports, asking them to review cases the QCs felt had possibly been in a status too long (for example, in status 02 longer than six months). Was this both proactive and reactive control—QCs using the former and counselors performing the latter?

8. One vocational rehabilitation professional urges counselors to review weekly the cases in their caseloads (Britten, 1981). I knew of none in the area office I observed who reviewed his or her caseload that often.

9. One intake worker in a welfare department noted that a holiday meant getting behind (Zimmerman, 1966: 260). That was often so for rehabilitation counselors.

10. In "getting" closures (and, to a lesser degree, plans) at the end of the fiscal year, counselors and the agency may also have sacrificed some quality. Almost thirty years ago, one rehabilitation professional commented that the counselor "knows that those who root for quality from July through January will be yelling 'Get those closures in' by April and May" (Johnston, 1957: 9-10). I've observed counselors either joking about holding cases until June in order to close them successfully or kidding a QC that at the end of the fiscal year he reviewed status 26 closures by turning away partially and glancing at them. This possible (slight) lowering of quality could be investigated by comparing the proportion of plans written at the end of the fiscal year (by those catching up) that became unsuccessful closures with those written at other times. Cases successfully closed at the end of the fiscal year (again, by those catching up) could be compared to those closed at other times by "independent" evaluators. There are other ways to check that possibility carefully, but I was not in a position to do so. However, one state-office professional casually agreed that

such probably did happen. (The professional also noted that high school clients might be better evaluated in November, when the crush of September was finished.) I take the professional's remarks to indicate that, being "professional," the professional realized that the working of human service agencies may not always be ideal because the agencies work within the real, imperfect world.

11. I suspect that at times counselors who met their goals early "saved" plans or closures until the beginning of the next fiscal year. They may have done so by holding onto them for a few days until turning them in, or, in handling other cases, they did not rush to complete them. In response to my questions, one counselor explained that the several closures he was finishing on July 1 could not have been turned in by the end of the previous fiscal year, and had he worked primarily on closures, he would have fallen behind on other responsibilities. However, he said that if you give the agency your goal and a few more, then you are doing fine. Was he implicitly acknowledging my hunch? I think so.

12. Some research and data (some of which are more informative than others, though none seem to be conclusive) suggest that the "more quickly clients move through the process the better their chances of becoming rehabilitated" (Willey, 1979: 155; Kunce et al., 1974; Tseng and Zerega, 1976; RSA, 1982b: 32). If there are delays in moving cases quickly, then many may be the counselors' responsibility, not just that of the applicants and clients. A study of "undue delays" in several southern and southwestern rehabilitation agencies indicated that counselors were more responsible than clients, the agency, "other," and the "environment." When the client's counselor was changed, "undue delay" almost always occurred (Cooper and Greenwood, 1975).

13. Compared to counselors nationwide, the counselors in the agency I investigated *seemed* to move cases quickly. Without controlling (or being able to control) for the severity of the disability/difficulty of the case (or whether the agency was a general vocational rehabilitation agency or one dealing strictly with blindness), the agency I observed established plans on about 55 percent of its successfully closed cases in a recent fiscal year in two months or less, kept approximately 37 percent of its successful closures from referral to closure nine months or less, and closed about 30 percent of its 26s within six months after putting the cases into plan status. The comparable figures nationwide were 52 percent, 24 percent, and 23 percent, respectively. A review of the agency in the late 1970s noted that, with a sense of "urgency" to process the cases quickly counselors did their casework, which may have led to some inappropriate decisions by counselors in thoroughly evaluating the clients' conditions. (In order to provide anonymity, I will not cite the sources for the above information.)

14. Rehabilitation professionals stress the need for avoiding delays and for moving cases in a "timely" manner through the rehabilitation process. One professional offers "practical" suggestions on how to "speed up" the processing of cases, such as "take an application and begin arranging diagnostics in the initial interview" instead of testing the referral's motivation by asking the referral to take the application home and return it (Willey, 1979: 156; Britten, 1981).

15. Counselors did not staff all such cases at the formal CDS meetings. Due to various reasons, such as missing the meeting because of other responsibilities or the need to obtain approval quickly, counselors staffed cases with their QC or colleagues outside the formal meetings. One counselor who worked at a school program no longer took "simple" cases, such as mentally retarded clients who were involved in the various special programs offered by the school and on whom relatively little money would be spent, to the CDS downtown. They were staffed with other professionals in the school rehabilitation program. The less transporting of folders the better, according to the counselor.

16. At times a counselor was designated as the leader of the staffing or was the leader by default when a QC or supervisor was not present. In the relatively few times a QC or

supervisor did not sit in on a CDS (even as an observer) *and* I recorded the length of the staffing and the number of cases staffed, I found that cases were staffed more quickly. Staffing took less than 2 minutes per case. When a counselor was the leader in a CDS, but supervisory personnel sat in (even sporadically), there was no significant difference in the amount of time it took to staff each case in comparison to when supervisory personnel were the leaders. It was perhaps because of the above-cited differences (and what those differences imply about the usefulness of staffings) that several years ago the agency instituted more formal staffings, though the form of staffings might still vary from area office to area office.

17. See Buckholdt and Gubrium (1979a: chap. 5; 1979b), Gubrium (1980a, 1980b), and Gubrium and Buckholdt (1982) for a discussion of how staffings are done. Among other issues, in a variety of settings they explore the professional image (world is taken for granted) and constructive image (the world is created) of staffings as well as three important techniques used by staffers to "do staffings": filling in, where staffers "construct meaningful understandings" of the clients, realizing, in which conjecture, interpretation, and "practical theorizing" become "solid stuff" (that is, fact); and glossing, by which staffers ignore or pass over "certain matters while attending to the business at hand" (Buckholdt and Gubrium 1979a: 180, 184). A difference between the staffings they explore and the CDS is that in the latter only the counselor in charge typically has much information about, and familiarity with, the case. Hence some of the techniques discussed by Buckholdt and Gubrium are not as fully realized in the CDS.

6

SPECIALTY CASELOADS

Detective work is often carried out in details: the juvenile detail, burglary detail, major crimes detail, vice squad, and the like. While the basic features of detective work—establishing a case, identifying a suspect, locating a suspect, "copping the suspect" (obtaining a confession), and disposing of the case—appear within the various details, the details themselves may vary. For example, vice squad detectives are generally much more proactive in obtaining cases to work than are those who work the burglary detail. What constitutes a "big case" in the juvenile detail, and therefore would be worked, might be quite "little" for major crimes. In fact, a "really" "big case" involving a juvenile, such as a robbery, might be given to the detectives in major crimes to work (Sanders, 1977: 43-44). And the investigations in major crimes tend to be much slower and more protracted than those carried out by detectives in burglary or juvenile (Sanders, 1977: 168). Through examining the details of the details, detective work comes alive. So it is for rehabilitation counselors and other human service professionals.
professionals.

Human service work is specialized, too. The person in need is parceled among the agencies that serve. The old, the young, the infirm, the uneducated, the poor, the "crazy," the criminal, the sick, and others are administered to by the appropriate agencies (Prottas, 1979: 3-4). And within those agencies, professionals specialize in their services. For example, within a department of social services or public welfare, the professionals are not just social workers, but intake workers, caseworkers, eligibility workers, CWS (Child Welfare Services) workers, and the like; often with further specialization within the various groups (Johnson, 1975: chap. 2; Prottas, 1979: 23). Rehabilitation counseling is specialized, too.

While rehabilitation counselors started as "jacks of all trades," in large part because in the early days of rehabilitation one agent was assigned to a territory with perhaps hundreds of thousands of people, they are increasingly becoming specialists (Warren, 1959; Wright, 1980: 59-60). One of the earliest bases for specialization was the disability of the client. Counselors worked with those who were visually impaired, mentally impaired, auditorily impaired, and so on, sometimes with further specialization within the particular disability (for example, blind versus those with "low" vision). In addition to specialists by disability ("horizontal" specialists), there were specialists by task ("vertical" specialization), who handled one function within the rehabilitation process (such as evaluation or job placement), and specialists in particular facilities or programs (such as school programs) with particular clients and concerns. Specialization was pursued, in part, to serve clients better, and it continues to be discussed in rehabilitation (Wright, 1980: 59-66).

In the area office I observed, many counselors did their rehabilitation work within specialty caseloads, whether those caseloads were identified formally as such or not. Specialization tended to be by disability or by the particular nature of the program/client. Approximately 40% of the active caseloads were officially designated as specialty caseloads. Several other counselors "unofficially" specialized to various degrees. Counselors specialized in school caseloads, those consisting of hearing-impaired individuals or of public offenders, and caseloads consisting primarily of persons with alcohol problems, those with primarily mental health problems, or those drawing workers compensation (due to a work-related injury). The basic features of rehabilitation work are found in these and other specialty caseloads (such as the defunct SSI and SSDI caseloads), though the specifics may vary.[1]

I examine four specialty caseloads: *hearing impaired, public offender, school,* and *alcoholic.* All of these are important within the agency for their services to a variety of individuals and important in helping the agency meet its goals.[2] In examining these caseloads, I do not explore every feature of rehabilitation previously discussed. Instead, I discuss several features that have special significance for the four caseloads. In doing so, I ground the general "doing" of rehabilitation work in the specifics of the specialty caseloads.

THE HEARING-IMPAIRED CASELOAD

In the area office one counselor served hearing-impaired clients. In addition to the on-the-job training other counselors received, the counselor who managed this specialty caseload participated in an intensive three-month training session at an out-of-state university that focused primarily on hearing impairments and, to a lesser extent, on vocational rehabilitation. During the training session, the counselor began to learn sign language, which she later used to converse with some of her clients. Thus, like detectives who receive special training because they handle particular kinds of cases, such as arson, counselors who specialized in serving clients with particular impairments may receive special training, too. In working the hearing-impaired caseload, the counselor faced many concerns such as working referrals, making a case, and providing substantial services.

Working Referrals

The counselor received referrals primarily from hearing aid dealers and otologists, and self-referrals from deaf individuals who were familiar with the agency from having attended the state residential school for the deaf, where the agency operated a rehabilitation program, or from being told by other members of the local deaf community. Due to a concern about receiving sufficient referrals to meet the caseload's goals, and in order to serve potential hearing-impaired clients more effectively, the counselor worked other referral sources, such as industrial audiologists and a local high school program for deaf students.

In working referrals, particularly hearing aid dealers, the counselor was concerned about maintaining professional, effective relations. To do so, the counselor needed to avoid offending the dealers by jeopardizing what the dealers took to be their rightful business. The dealers' business would be jeopardized when individuals whom they referred to the vocational rehabilitation agency were not sent back to them when a hearing aid was to be purchased, when the agency did not distribute its "hearing aid business" (their purchases of aids for clients who had not been referred by a dealer) evenly, and when recommended services were not fully provided at a reasonable price by the agency.

To avoid antagonizing dealers, the counselor attempted, when possible, to inform the dealer (or another referral source) if the dealer's client did contact the agency, and, if so, how that contact turned out. (Unless the dealer had informed the counselor of a referral, it would be almost impossible to let the dealer know when a dealer's client did not contact the agency.) By doing so, if the dealers' clients were not appearing for appointments, or if they were not eligible for the agency's services, then the "loss of business" would not be attributed to the agency. When referrals were eligible for services, one of which was a hearing aid, the counselor attempted to make sure the client was sent back to the dealer who had referred the individual (or who had previously served the individual). As the counselor explained:

> Well, the main problem that seems to come up is that sometimes, if a client comes in referred by one dealer in town, . . . we honor that referral. If they have worked with another dealer in the past sometimes that causes a conflict. . . . I always try to find out who they [the clients] used in the past, which dealer, so they won't cause all these problems because they [the dealers] get upset, and I guess I can understand that, if you send them to somebody else to get a hearing aid . . . [and] they have been using . . . one service in town in the past. And I asked her [speaking of a client] and she said . . . [that] she had never used anybody in town, and so . . . I sent her to a certain dealer, and it just so happened that the dealer called me back and said, "Oh, we have worked with her before." . . . I just got lucky then. I could have very well sent her to somebody else . . . and that could have caused a lot of problems, but it just so happened that I got lucky and sent her back to one that she had used before. She didn't remember, and a lot of them don't remember or they say . . . [that] it doesn't matter, and . . . I have no way of knowing.

When a client had not been referred by a dealer, but the counselor intended to purchase a hearing aid as part of the plan of services, then the "business" was "spread around" to dealers with whom the agency had a contract. Finally, the counselors tried to clear up any misunderstandings the dealers had concerning the payment schedule the agency followed, the counselor's inability to provide aids for individuals who were not economically eligible, and the like. These misunderstandings might be addressed when they arose or when contracts between the agency and the dealers were renewed. However, according to the counselor, some dealers were probably not referring their clients to the agency due to previous misunderstandings and dissatisfaction.

Making a Case

While establishing hearing-impaired referrals' eligibility for the agency's services was no longer particularly problematic to the counselor, two issues were significant: eliciting the vocational problems the referrals experienced due to their hearing impairments and making certain that what the agency could provide was satisfactory to the referral. During the initial interview, the counselor attemped to elicit the ways in which the referral's hearing impairment was a problem to the referral. The counselor focused on employment, but not exclusively. While some referrals had a "laundry list" of problems they recounted to the counselor, others simply said that they could not hear. According to the counselor, these referrals, sincere in their answers, probably thought that the counselor was "crazy" for asking such an obvious question. In such cases the counselor elicited problems through specific questioning of the referrals. Did the referral need to ask people to repeat their messages? Did these people become angry at being asked to do so? Did the referral avoid going places because of the hearing impairment? Did the referral worry that the impairment might worsen? Did the referral feel self-conscious about a hearing aid? Even those who recounted a "laundry list" of problems could be prompted with questions concerning the effect of their hearing impairments on their jobs and/ or interactions with others. These and similar questions were asked to substantiate that the disability was a vocational handicap. The referrals' responses were documented in the R-1 notes and mentioned in the evaluation summaries when plans of services were developed.

The counselor developed these "eliciting" questions based on personal experience with a hearing impairment, her clients' experiences, and the training she received during the three-month training session. These questions, listed on a sheet of paper, were now infrequently referred to as the counselor had developed more experience. However, the questions still proved useful.

When establishing eligibility, the counselor was concerned to make certain the referral would be satisfied with what the agency would be able to provide. The issue was "tangibles," specifically hearing aids (and possibly corrective surgery). Many referrals wanted something tangible from the agency: medical follow-up, work clothes, surgery, or the like. Hearing-impaired referrals were no different. Some wanted the agency to purchase them a hearing aid or provide corrective surgery. If they were not economically eligible for those services (that is, they could afford to pay for them according to the agency's criteria), then they might not be interested in what the agency could provide, such as guidance and counseling. Therefore, based on experience, the counselor determined the economic eligibility of referrals whom she felt would be primarily interested in tangibles *before* she conducted the bulk of the initial interview and filled in the application. Such referrals were those who were currently employed but who were experiencing difficulties due to their impairments. Others who were unemployed, whether or not economically eligible for the agency's assistance in purchasing a hearing aid, could be provided job placement assistance as well as counseling and guidance. Thus, in establishing eligibility, the counselor needed to elicit the problems experienced by the referrals as well as determine that what the referrals wanted from the agency could be provided by the agency.

Substantial Services

In working the hearing-impaired caseloads, the counselor mentally separated the caseload into three categories: those who were deaf, those who were "hard of hearing" and without a job, and those who were "hard of hearing" and employed. Each category was seen as involving different problems to be dealt with and services to render. The counselor explained:

> Well, the three categories that I kind of divide it up into: those deaf clients, which most of them are going to need maybe some evaluation or some kind of adjustment services in job placement and then a lot of follow-up. . . . . Another category would be my hard-of-hearing clients who . . . may or may not need evaluation or adjustment services that would also need job placement, and the third category would be the hard-of-hearing clients who . . . maybe are already working on the job but need some assistance with their hearing and coping with their hearing loss.

During the course of their work, counselors who worked specialty caseloads may have specialized even further.

The counselor found that cases involving hard-of-hearing clients were easier to handle. They involved purchasing a hearing aid and counseling and guiding the clients about their hearing losses and their aids. Many of them were already employed. Cases involving deaf clients were more difficult but also more rewarding. The counselor was more directly involved in job placement with deaf clients: setting up job interviews and preparing them for those interviews, counseling them regarding good work habits (for example, being punctual or informing employers when they would be late or absent), interpreting for the clients during the interviews and during orientation when they obtained a job, and perhaps even answering for them in interviews when it seemed that they would answer inappropriately.

As the agency reduced its "bill-paying" cases, providing substantial services became a concern to counselors. The counselor who handled the hearing-impaired caseload was initially concerned that her IWRPs for her "hard-of-hearing" clients would be accepted by the QCs. In order to not have plans "kicked back" because they looked only like "bill-paying," the counselor detailed more clearly on the plans what services she was intending to provide, other than purchasing a hearing aid. During the few years the counselor had worked with the agency, she had developed and modified a list of "counseling areas for the hearing impaired." The list was based on what her clients had shared with her and on her own study in the area of hearing impairment. Unlike her list of "eliciting" questions, this counseling list was employed constantly as the counselor developed plans and served clients. Counseling areas included psychological areas, such as feelings of isolation, withdrawal tendencies, and concerns about cosmetic aspects of the hearing aid, technical areas, such as maintenance of and adjustment to the aid, and conservation of residual hearing. These and similar counseling areas were emphasized so that the cases did not simply become "bill-paying" cases.[3] Through successfully working referral sources, making a case, and providing substantial services, the counselor maintained a productive hearing-impaired caseload.

THE PUBLIC OFFENDER CASELOAD[4]

While there was only one officially designated public offender caseload in the area office, several counselors who handled general caseloads also had responsibility for men and women who were released from prison and were to be served by the agency. Furthermore, during the course of my research several counselors had responsibility for the officially designated public offender caseload. Therefore, several counselors had experience in working with public offender clients. The bulk of my discussion, however, focuses on the counselors who handled the male public offenders. To those working a public offender caseload, the nature of the caseload, the "nature" of the clients (and how that affected rehabilitation work), and "sugar money" (the "tangibles" received by the clients, such as clothes, money, and tools), were important, interrelated concerns.

The Nature of the Caseload

The public offender caseload was a high-volume, relatively quick-turnover caseload.[5] It was assigned the highest goal of successful closures in the state. Whoever managed it was expected to produce. To produce, however, did not involve the full range of rehabilitation detective work as often as did the other caseloads. Most cases the counselors worked arrived in plan status, the plan having been developed and much of the guidance and counseling having been provided by vocational rehabilitation counselors who worked in the correctional facilities. While the counselor was responsible for developing a relatively small number of plans during the fiscal year (about half as many as most other counselors), that responsibility was seen as much less important than producing successful closures. The field counselors' task was to conclude cases successfully.

Contacts with the public offender clients typically were fewer and of a slightly different nature than what occurred on other caseloads. The initial contact by the field counselor generally was not with a referral, but with a client who had already been provided some sevices while in prison. That initial contact usually occurred approximately one week before the clients were to be released (in a batch) from a prerelease center of the state's correctional system. Counselors throughout the state who handled public offenders met at the prerelease center, chatted with one another, were provided lists of clients who were locating in their territories and folders for their clients, and then dispersed to individual rooms to see their clients. During the short, few-minutes-long conversations, the counselors questioned and confirmed where the clients woud be living when they left, with whom they would be living, whether or not they had jobs arranged and, if not, what their interests were, and whether they were being released on parole or "maxing out" (had served their full sentences and, therefore, were being released without any conditions placed on them). The counselors for the local area office explained to their clients that when they were released they would be seen at the "old" downtown office where a "small" ($35) maintenance check would be provided. The check would help them pay some of their expenses until they obtained jobs or received their first paychecks. It would also help them pay for transportation while looking for jobs. A second maintenance check, along with a modest amount of work clothes and/or tools, if needed, would also be provided when the client obtained work. The counselors briefly advised clients to "stay out of trouble," follow through, address their alcohol problems if they had them, and be "straight" with the counselors. As one counselor often told clients, "Don't tell me you're going to do something if you're not going to do it."

When the clients were released, generally the next week, the counselors met them at the downtown office, which was more convenient for the clients than the new office "across the river" in an adjacent city. During this brief contact the major transaction was the provision of the first maintenance check to the clients, though discussion between the counselors and clients might center on living arrangements, jobs, keeping out of trouble, and other immediate concerns. Whether the clients' cases were closed as successfully rehabilitated or not depended in part on whether or not there were additional contacts. For many clients, these two contacts—the first in the prerelease center, the second when they were released—were the only ones with the field counselors. If so, the cases were not closed as successfully rehabilitated.

Whether the cases were closed successfully or not, the out-of-pocket expenses for the cases were relatively modest. Medical evaluations were performed by the correctional department as part of the management of their prisoners, and psychological evaluations were conducted by the rehabilitation agency's staff. Maintenance money and, where needed, work clothes and tools (typically the minimum necessary hand tools, according to one counselor) might amount to $100 to a few hundred dollars. A high-volume, relatively inexpensive caseload was important to an agency that wanted to serve many people.

The "Nature" of the Clients

Unlike general caseloads, in which counselors worked with clients with a wide variety of disabilities, those who handled public offender caseloads worked within a much narrower range. Public offenders typically became eligible based on a psychological disability, in particular, an antisocial personality disorder. Less clinically, though perhaps more descriptively, field counselors viewed many, though certainly not all, of their public offender clients as often irresponsible individuals who would lie to and con the counselor. The clients expected something for nothing. They were belligerent, demanding, and usually ungrateful.

Clients' actions often served as (further) proof of their "nature." Clients who claimed never to have received the maintenance check in order to avoid paying their room and board at a halfway house for ex-offenders, those who "took the money and ran," never to be seen again, clients who conned the counselors into believing they had jobs in order to receive the second maintenance check, those who worked a few days or weeks and then vanished ("two-week" people, as described by one counselor), and the majority, whom counselors had to contact continually because they did not contact the counselors and who showed little appreciation for what had been done for them, proved continually to the counselors, through their actions, their highly unconventional nature. For example, the following incident was described to me several times, in humor and disgust, and served as an example of the nature of public offender clients:

> One client arranged for a friend to stand by at a telephone so that, when the counselor called to confirm the client's employment, the client's friend answered the phone and confirmed that the client was working. A day or two later the counselor called back and learned that the phone was located in a party shop, pool hall, or "something like that." The client had conned the counselor out of the second maintenance check.

"Of course," as noted by one counselor, the offenders' nature was part of their problem, leading to troubles with the law and troubles for their rehabilitation counselors.

Because of the nature of public offender clients (according to the counselors), counselors were active in safeguarding the integrity of their services. However, they were not always successful. The public offender caseload produced not only a large number of 26s but also of 28s. Nevertheless, counselors attempted to safeguard the integrity of their services in various ways. One counselor told public offender clients bluntly that fellow clients were often irresponsible and asked the clients not to lie to him. Although it was not clear that such counseling was effective, at least it indicated to the clients that the counselor was not naive about what could happen. When maintenance checks were distributed, counselors had clients sign for them so they could not claim later to have been shortchanged. When clients claimed to be working for friends or relatives, counselors became suspicious and might attempt to check more carefully before issuing a second maintenance check. Experience had taught them that lesson. By talking with family members or "check[ing] a little bit more and maybe mak[ing] an extra contact somewhere or other," counselors began to attempt to verify their client's employment because their client's word was becoming increasingly questioned.

Counselors were also concerned about protecting their own and the agency's reputations. Based on experience with clients who conned them and angered employers by quitting soon after beginning work, and based on their scant familiarity with the clients, counselors were reluctant to put their names "on the line" when placing the clients. A counselor who worked the officially designated public offender caseload had very few clients whom he would recommend to employers. As he explained:

> I don't have close contact with them [the public offender clients], and these people are somewhat unreliable, and I just do not feel comfortable in going and telling an employer that I have someone who is reliable. . . . What I'll do when [I] talk to someone, I say, "Well, you know some of his [the client's] background. I can't guarantee that he'll stay with you on and on," or that sort of thing, you know. I try to be straight with the people [the employers]. Otherwise, they get to where they won't talk to us about it. Matter of fact, I've had one hang up on me one time anyway.

Guarded recommendations, or none at all, helped safeguard the counselor's and agency's reputations from the possibly irresponsible behavior of the clients.

To protect the agency's services (as well as extend the agency's help), counselors often had to track clients. Even successful cases often involved the counselors' contacting the clients rather than the clients' contacting the counselors (unless the former wanted something tangible). Tracking public offender clients was beset with difficulties similar to those faced by other counselors, though perhaps the difficulties were more forcefully felt in the case of public offenders. Home visits were a frequent necessity when one worked with public offenders, though it was not always certain where "home" was. Clients who "maxed out," and therefore did not need to report to parole officers, were seen as particularly problematic. They had even less reason than the others to stay in touch and stay around. Those who were from outside the area but claimed to be relocating in the area once they were released from prison often left after a few weeks. More and better references would be helpful in tracking clients, but clients were sometimes unwilling or unable to provide them. If the parole officers did not know where the clients were, then it would certainly be difficult for the counselors to know. Family members and neighbors might not be particularly helpful. Either they did not know where the client was (which, in regard to family members, struck one counselor as incredible) or they refused to say. To family members and neighbors, the counselor, a stranger and often of a different race than they, might be the police or some other official, such as a collection agent, which only meant trouble. Consequently, one counselor made a point of introducing himself as an employee of the vocational rehabilitation agency in order to allay the family's and neighbor's suspicions. In one home visit he told the sister of his client that he was not looking to "get" the client. Unfortunately, clients were often not "gotten" (found).

"Sugar Money"

"Sugar money" was a key to the concerns, difficulties, and successes of public offender caseloads. Sugar money was what one rehabilitation professional facetiously suggested the maintenance checks, work clothes, and tools be called. They were the tangibles that sweetened the intangible, and less sought, guidance and counseling. Without the sugar money, counselors claimed that successful closures would decrease dramatically. I suspect they were correct, but then unsuccessful closures might have decreased too, as offenders who were involved in the program solely for the sugar money decreased their participation.

Sugar money was both a blessing and a curse for the counselors. With it, counselors were able to attract many offenders to the program. With strings attached to the second maintenance check, the work clothes, and tools, the sugar money became a small leverage in getting clients back to work.[6] However, in conjunction with the nature of the clients, sugar money led to many of the difficulties faced by the counselors. Counselors' concerns with clients who "took the money and ran," with being conned out of a second maintenance check, with ex-offenders who were not clients but wanted a check anyway, and with clients who conned halfway houses out of room and board all involved sugar money.

The significance of sugar money in public offender caseloads led to a broader concern for the counselors, too. Did the services provided to the public offenders make a substantial difference or not? When first meeting the offenders at the prerelease center, one counselor told them that what the agency provided was "just a little bit of help" to ease the transition from prison to the outside world. That counselor and another wondered how helpful that "little bit" was to the public offenders. For these counselors, who did not provide as much guidance and counseling to their clients as did many other counselors, whose job often seemed to involve primarily dispensing sugar money (though other services were certainly provided, too) and tracking wayward clients, and who experienced many failures as well as successes, concern about their impact was understandable. Perhaps more so than by counselors on any other caseload, the "human service" aspect of rehabilitation work was questioned by those who serviced public offender caseloads.

THE SCHOOL CASELOAD

Public school caseloads constituted the majority of specialty caseloads in the area office I studied. Almost one-third of the caseloads in the office were designated as public school caseloads. Several other counselors also handled students as part of their general caseloads. Due to the number of counselors involved with public school students and to the relative proportion of the area office's total production goals assigned to them, public school caseloads were important within the agency.

Typically housed in a high school or other school facility, the public school programs were staffed by counselors, casework assistants, a project supervisor who supervised the program in addition to having caseload responsibilities, an evaluator who assessed the students' vocational interests and skills, and work adjustment personnel when the program had a workshop where students developed appropriate work skills. Because of the nature of school caseloads, counselors needed to establish and maintain working relations with the students and to channel them toward appropriate vocational objectives.

The Nature of the Caseload

School caseloads served students (or former students), usually between the ages of 16 and 21. Some who were being sponored in colleges and universities might be older. Until several years ago, students as young as 14 could be served by the counselors. However, the agency decided that, because the legal minimum age for employment was 16, it was difficult to justify working with students who could not legally be employed for several years. There was no existing reasonable expectation that a 14-year-old would go to work. Further, services were being "watered down," and evaluations were becoming out of date in working with the students over such a long period. With changes in the agency's policy, counselors were then allowed to open cases on students who were 15½, but not to begin to serve them until they turned 16.

While students with a wide variety of disabilities were seen, those who were mentally retarded or had emotional problems (often diagnosed as adolescent adjustment reaction) dominated the caseloads. Therefore, the caseloads were not greatly affected by the recent changes of the agency away from "paying a bill." Nor did they tend to be costly caseloads. Counseling and guidance, work adjustment, and job placement assistance were "no-cost" services (that is, they were provided by agency personnel in agency facilities without being purchased). One school counselor's budget was one-fifth of a general counselor's budget, although both worked out of the same office and served approximately the same geographical territory. The school counselor's goals were lower than the general counselor's, but still much more than one-fifth of the general counselor's.

Referrals to the rehabilitation counselors came from many sources in the schools. Teachers and guidance counselors, particularly those who worked with students who received special services because of their disabilities, were important referral sources. One school project supervisor noted:

> If you try to develop a good relationship there with the guidance people and the teacher, then you won't have any problems getting referrals. Matter of fact, you'll have as many as you can handle.

Students who were satisfied with the assistance they had received might refer classmates. Secretaries who had "picked up on problems" or administrators in charge of discipline sometimes referred students. Some counselors reviewed students' school records for indications that students might be well served by the agency, and some became aware of potential clients when notified of students' suspensions or excessive absences.

Counselors also distributed a physical condition survey form for students to check. Approximately forty "conditions," such as "crossed eyes," "severe asthma," "frequent stomach pains," "numbness in any area," and "loss of limb," were listed. By questioning the students in person, the counselors determined whether or not those paper referrals were worth pursuing. Some students did not recall completing the survey. Perhaps a friend had signed their name to one. Others had not been serious when they had completed it. And still others had completed the survey in good faith, but, upon questioning, the counselor decided the students did not need the agency's services: skin allergies were causing no problems; a scar on a leg posed no vocational obstacle; a vision problem was "just lazy eye"; or an ulcer due to "greasy food" had cleared up (see Chapter 3).

Students had little if any knowledge of vocational rehabilitation, had not sought out the counselors, and, because the counselors were typically based in the schools, may have mistaken the counselors for school personnel. Thus, in contrast to many adult referrals, student referrals were much less educated about the rehabilitation agency (and human service agencies in general) and had shown less initiative to be involved in the agency's programs. They were not necessarily reluctant referrals—though some were—as much as they were indifferent referrals. As one school project supervisor explained:

> nine times out of the ten those referrals came by way-of . . . the guidance counselor or a teacher, and the student really didn't know that much about VR and probably could have cared less about what we did. . . . that's no blame to them because we were in the school. They looked at us as school people, not VR people, and it was very difficult to explain to a lot of them, you know. It was just that situation . . . you could easily just sit back and probably say that 90 percent were not interested. Just close the case on them, you know. Really not do any follow-up. But to me that's really not meeting the needs there.

Students also typically had little work experience and often no well-developed and realistic vocational objectives. To one school project supervisor, the students' lack of experience made school caseloads "probably the most difficult of all":

> You have nothing to build on. When you have an adult that's been in the labor force for ten or eleven or twenty years, you got a variety of job experience. Even though a lot of . . . [them] may not be able to return to the same job, some of the skills are still transferable. But with young people, you basically start . . . from scratch. You don't have anything to build on. . . . Most of the kids we work with here have never had a job. They may have . . . done a little yard work or in summers . . . maybe a little city job or something like that, but real . . . job-experience-type jobs. . . .

Particularly since the great bulk of my caseload are the mentally retarded class, they really are at a terrible disadvantage because they don't know anything about work.

Others changed their vocational interests "based on peer pressures, the hottest thing going among (their) peers." And others had "unrealistic" objectives. As one counselor noted:

We have one student that wants to be a movie star. That is completely unrealistic here. He is a very slow learner. It's just not practical, and that's what he wants to do. He is going to have to make up his mind and realize he is not going to be able to go to Hollywood and be a movie star.

School caseloads involved youthful clients, who had little or no knowledge about the rehabilitation agency, often relatively little commitment to the agency because the agency had approached them rather than their having approached the agency, and little or no work history. There was a "world of difference" between school caseloads and general caseloads, according to one counselor who had worked both. Out of those "differences" came the necessity to establish and maintain working relations with the students and to channel them toward appropriate vocational objectives.

Establishing and Maintaining Working Relations

Students were naive referrals. They had little, if any, understanding of the agency and often little, if any, awareness of why they were being referred to the rehabilitation counselor. The counselor's task was to educate the students about the agency in such a way that students who were potential clients would become interested in the agency. Once educated, the students' motivation needed to be sustained. A working relationship had be established and maintained.

The counselors attempted to sell their services to the students. Those who referred the students could help by informing the students why they were being referred and by "playing up the angle as far as providing services to them on the placement end," according to one counselor. The counselors themselves indicated to the students what they might be able to do for them: medical evaluation and follow-up, vocational evaluation, career planning, possible sponsorship to postsecondary training, and assistance in obtaining a job (perhaps a part-time or summer job and later a full-time job upon graduation). One counselor explained:

> I always try to do what I could to fit, if this makes any sense, to fit the client or referral into VR, in other words, try to pick a part of what we do and match it up with the need of the referral. . . . If I could do that, sometimes I could reach the person, and the person would become interested in that particular thing. For example, if I had a client who wanted . . . to go to [a technical college] . . . to be a machine operator, I might could explain to him or her that I could get some information for them from [the technical college] . . . and if there would be a possibility that we would help them with some training, pay for some training possibly. I always had to speak in possibilities and "ifs" and all that with them, no commitment, but if I could reach a real interested area with a referral, a lot of times they would come around and show some interest.

In establishing a working relationship, counselors were often concerned about not setting the students apart from their classmates. While the agency's mandate was to serve individuals with vocationally *handicapping disabilities,* several counselors tried not to emphasize that the referred students were handicapped or disabled. Instead, did the students have a "problem" that interfered with their school activities and home life and might later interfere with employment? If so, then the counselor could help the students with their problems, particularly as they related to work. One mentioned to students that he was like a second counselor (in addition to the guidance counselor), so that students would see him in a much more routine, less threatening way. Later, when rapport had been established between the counselor and the youth, terms such as "handicap" or "disability" might be used. If the terms "handicap" and "disability" were used from the outset, the counselor did not dwell on them. Rather, the counselor focused attention on how the agency could assist the youths, particularly with career choices and employment. Psychological evaluations might be referred to as tests to see where the students felt "unsure" of themselves or for "getting to know more about" them. Jokes, compliments, and mildly self-disparaging remarks (such as "I'm not very good in math either") were used to put the students at ease. Thus counselors attempted to establishd a working relationship with the naive referrals by selling themselves and their agency to the youths and by trying to keep them at ease by not dwelling on their handicaps or disabilities.

By establishing a working relationship with a student, counselors attempted to develop the youth's interest in the agency and its services.

Maintaining interest and involvement was a concern, too. One counselor noted:

> You can set up ten appointments and you might not even see two [students] at most. . . .
>
> [Is that a difficulty working with high school students?]
>
> Yes, because . . . kids, well they are kids. They don't follow through as opposed to adults.

In attempting to maintain the youths' motivation, counselors collectively used a mixture of counseling and guidance and tangibles. Counseling and guidance might include being a "big brother or father figure or whatever" to the youths or "twist[ing] their arms or prod[ding] them or whatever to get them to follow through." Social workers assigned to the family from the social services department might be asked to help students keep their appointments. Sometimes the assistance of parents was sought. On one home visit a counselor asked the client's mother to "talk up" the daughter's evaluation, which the counselor was arranging. As another counselor noted:

> You had to do a lot of extra things, like contacting parents and try to get them to help with some of the follow-up that the student was to do with us.

However, unlike detectives in a West Coast juvenile detail, who often saw parents as allies in doing their job (parents could be told of their child's trouble and discipline left to them; Sanders, 1977: 144-147), rehabilitation counselors did not have those allies as often as they would have liked. Without parental consent, counselors could not even work with the students. Too often, however, consent was all the counselors received. One counselor said of the parents of inner-city clients:

> So very few of the parents really care, you know . . . just very few of them really are even concerned or even know about the program. . . . You can tell them about it, but they'll say, "Oh, that sounds good." And that's the last you hear from them. . .
>
> [Does that make it difficult for you to do your job? With the parents not giving you their support?]
>
> Well, [for] most . . . the family is not intact . . . don't know where the father is, . . . might have seven or eight other kids . . . living under [social services] support . . . there's not any parental supervision there, and there is not anybody you can call and say, "Hey, Johnnie is acting up. Can you do something about it?" . . . There is a lot of apathy there in the parents. So we don't . . . really get much support. We do occasionally, but not too much.

Calls and letters to the parents did not always develop that support either.

Personal contact with selected students during the summer or with those who, no longer attending their high schools, were waiting to enter a special school for students who had experienced difficulties in "regular" schools helped to maintain the youths' interest and involvement. It also demonstrated the counselors' continuing concern with the youths. One counselor described youthful clients who were waiting to enter that special school:

> There would be kind of a vacuum period there where they would not be in high school or not doing anything, and their parents would be working, and they would be at home and a lot of just not doing anything. And it took a lot . . . of maintaining contact with that person, mak[ing] sure they didn't fall by the wayside and lose interest in going to school. And in dealing with that, I try to . . . have them . . . contact me, sometimes twice a week, come by to talk with me.

Because the youths "wanted time and they wanted attention," the counselor's personal contact was important in maintaining the youths' involvement in the rehabilitation process. Like detectives who work a juvenile detail, school rehabilitation counselors realized that more personal and less bureaucratic attention was needed in working with youthful clients (Sanders, 1977: 144-147).

Counseling and guidance through personal contact, however, was not always enough. It was difficult at times to maintain the youths' motivation because the payoff (a job) might be several years in the future. Tangibles could prove helpful. The special school, which provided another opportunity for those who were not making it in their high schools, was one tangible; a summer job was another. Perhaps the most immediate tangible was the work adjustment programs that were operated by the vocational rehabilitation school projects. Work, contracted by the project supervisor to be done for local businesses, provided students the opportunity to develop work skills and habits and to earn money on a piece-rate basis. Those earnings were a "big motivator," according to one counselor:

> The students are paid on a piece-rate basis. And that in itself is a motivation to keep them working, rather than playing. Sometimes a student will say, "Hey, so and so made more." The first thing they do when they get their check, they start comparing them. We ask them not to, but they are going to go around a corner and compare checks. And some of them say, "Hey, so and so made more than I did. Why?" "He worked while you were down there talking. Remember the other day . . . ?" This has an

effect on them. It is a teaching tool. They do remember and they do learn. So it helps to make them work better. . . . This brings them around to realizing, as much as anything else, they have to work. They do have to be able to function in order to be able to get out.

The work adjustment program may also have helped motivate students to follow through (in evaluations) in order to "get in" the program. The same counselor found that at another school for which he was responsible, but where no work adjustment program was available, a small, but significant, percentage of the referred youths would "not get a general medical" "because the students there [did] not have work adjustment to help motivate them." And for some of the students who had access to work adjustment but did not take it seriously, the difficulty in finding jobs may have been the more successful (but perhaps too late) "teaching tool."

Channeling Toward a Vocation

Due to a lack of work experience, student clients often changed their vocational goals and/or held unrealistic goals. As one counselor noted, "You might have them come in and tell you they want to be a truck driver. Next day they might come in and say an engineer." Or, a youth with an IQ test score of 59 might want to be a registered nurse, and another with an IQ of "80 or 75, something like that," might want to be a lawyer or doctor. Unlike many other counselors who handled adults with work experience, school rehabilitation counselors could not depend on their client's prior work experiences in deciding on and making a commitment to vocational objectives. Instead, they used other strategies to try to channel their clients toward a vocation.

A vocational evaluation conducted by the school project's evaluator, which assessed the clients' skills and interests, was standard procedure. During the evaluation the evaluator might counsel the clients about their vocational goals. Results of the evaluation were shared with the clients. Where an objective could not be developed due to the limited skills of the clients, an extended evaluation, up to eighteen months long, might be used. However, after evaluation, some still held to unrealistic objectives. Experience, whether in extended evaluation or when the student began to "get out and taste the job market," might lead some to realize that their vocational objectives would need to be changed. As one counselor remarked:

Time does a lot for us. So you may not be able to come up with a concrete objective that he [the client] would agree with. We will go ahead maybe and do an extended evaluation, and we can keep him in there for eighteen months. And during that period of time he will do some work. And . . . usually they come around and say, "Hey I realize I can't do this."

Channeling the youth toward a related, but less demanding, objective might be a successful strategy. The client with an IQ score of 59 might be urged to "do something like nurse's assistant" instead of aiming to be an RN. However, counselors did not want to confront their youthful clients bluntly with their lack of skill and unrealistic goals. To do so might be damaging to the client and self-defeating for the counselor. As one counselor said:

Don't try to convince the child that, "No you don't have these skills." I won't approach them like that and try to break his ego or anything.

Instead, by focusing on what the youths could do, showing them the requirements of their unrealistic objectives, and allowing them to realize for themselves that their skills were not appropriate for their vocational choices, counselors more subtly "backed" their clients down to more obtainable vocational objectives.

As the clients' interests and opportunities changed, the counselors had to be ready with amendments to justify those changes. While some justifications may be difficult according to one counselor (see Chapter 4), due to the often limited skills of the clients, the vocational changes were often within a limited range: brick mason instead of carpenter, or food service worker instead of office worker. Thus, according to the same counselor, in order to handle the changes in vocational objectives, it was "just a matter of additional paperwork, really." Basic services did not need to be changed. Other counselors were not quite so sanguine about the vocational changes and amendments (and possibly related changes in services) needed to justify them. Nevertheless, through evaluation, some initial experience with work, redirection toward related fields, and amendments, counselors were able to channel youthful clients toward vocations.

THE ALCOHOLIC CASELOAD

While not an officially designated specialty caseload, one caseload in the area office involved primarily those with drinking (and, to a much lesser extent, drug) problems. While other counselors handled those with drinking problems (and were more likely to keep such clients as "bill-paying" cases "dried-up"), the counselor in charge of this caseload specialized in serving those with alcohol problems. The caseload had not originally been established as an unofficial specialty caseload, but, through development, it became one. The counselor's development of referral sources, which led to an unofficial specialty caseload, the emphasis on referrals' commitment to addressing their problems, concern with "running with cases," and the routinization in working cases were striking features of the alcoholic caseload.

Developing an Alcoholic Caseload

When the counselor took over the alcoholic caseload, it was a general caseload, with one referral source being a local alcohol and drug abuse center (to that limited extent it was already an alcoholic caseload). However, because of the center's procedures, which required that all referrals from the center go through one drug abuse counselor before they reached the rehabilitation counselor, very few referrals reached the latter. While that drug abuse counselor was on vacation, the referrals increased dramatically (to ten in two weeks), but declined (to one a week at most) when the counselor returned to work. The drug abuse counselor eventually left the center, with referrals then increasing to approximately twelve per month for "quite a while." By informing other drug abuse counselors that he could help their clients in ways other than arranging for long-term treatment at two state facilities, the rehabilitation counselor gradually developed the alcohol and drug abuse center into a productive referral source.

The rehabilitation counselor capitalized on happenstance in developing his other major referral source. As mentioned in Chapter 5, at a local hospital the counselor ran into a federal rehabilitation counselor who worked at local federal hospital. The federal counselor mentioned that he needed some help in serving the patients in an addiction treatment program. After several months, the referral source began to produce. The counselor relied not only on the patients referred to him by the federal counselor, but also screened the patients actively to determine whether or not they were interested in services. With the help of the federal counselor, the hospital became a productive referral source. In the previous year, only one case from the hospital had been opened. The counselor opened 55 the first year and more than 60 in just 9 months of the following year. Other referral sources were also developed in connection with various units of the hospital: one dealing with psychiatric patients, which the counselor who specialized in alcoholic cases initially handled, another with those who had physical problems, and a fourth drawing referrals from the nursing home of the hospital, which was later combined with the third into one caseload.

As the rehabilitation counselor's two primary referral sources began to produce, his caseload became an unofficial specialty caseload involving those with alcohol problems. As he noted, "Most anybody who deals with any type of alcohol problems knows me and [can] call and feel comfortable in making referrals to me." The counselor stopped working a small territory that had been part of the caseload. He gave up the psychiatric patients to a fellow counselor. Months later, as his referrals remained high and as other counselors needed some, he was asked to share his referral source at the drug and alcohol abuse center with a colleague. With "too much" success came the necessity to share some of it with others.

The referral sources were "good." They provided many cases, often "good" ones. Because the sources were medical facilities, medical evaluations were readily available, especially when the counselor became an unpaid consultant so that he could photocopy the clients' records at the federal hospital instead of depending on someone else to do it. With medical records readily available, plans could be developed with little delay, an important consideration to the counselor. The need for counseling and guidance was apparent (and was provided by both the referral sources and the counselor). Cases were typically inexpensive. With the medical evaluations being provided through the two referral sources, with many of the services being provided by the referral sources and the state treatment facilities, and with the referrals being adults who typically had previous work experience that lessened the need for training, the cost of the cases to the agency was relatively modest: perhaps a maintenance check and some work clothes and tools, if needed. Further, the counselor received relatively few "street alcoholics," those who lived and drank on the streets. According to the counselor, those alcoholics would "almost have to . . . [make] a commitment that would change their lifestyle." Few apparently did. Those street alcoholics who were referred to the counselor often did not follow through. They screened themselves out by not reappearing to have applications taken. However, even with few street alcoholics on the caseload, the counselor expected to lose about one-third of the referrals by their not following through. While that was frustrating, it was "just one of the things . . . [to be] expected" (expected by supervisory personnel, too). The high volume of referrals and the availability of medical records was compensation for the "pretty unstable" situation of many of the referrals (such as no well-established address or few family ties). Through persistance and by capitalizing on happenstance, the counselor had developed a productive, unofficial specialty caseload for himself and referral sources for several of his colleagues.

Commitment

A cornerstone of the counselor's philosophy was the need for those with drinking problems to make a commitment to stop drinking and address their problems through treatment. Referrals and clients must be sober. If not, then the counselor would rarely take an application, talk with the individual, or continue the job-search process. Through experience, the counselor found that those who were drunk did not benefit from what he or others could offer. For example, the state treatment facilities required individuals to be sober for 72 hours before being admitted. Because the counselor felt that those who were willing to admit they needed help should receive it immediately, the counselor used to apologize for that rule. However, he later came to believe that the individual with a drinking problem would benefit little from the program and would be a disruptive influence on the others in the program unless he or she was sober.

But "drying out" was not enough. Instead, being involved in a treatment program, whether one operated by the federal hospital, the two state facilities, the local alcohol and drug abuse center, or Alcoholics Anonymous, was an indication of the alcoholics' sincerity to do something about their problem. However, those who had gone to several treatment facilities in succession and were still drinking showed bad faith. Perhaps they needed to "hurt more" before they were able to make a sincere commitment. Consequently, before beginning to work with such clients again, the counselor might let them "cool their heels" until he felt they were ready to address their problems seriously. Or he might "make a deal" whereby the individuals must be sober when they saw a drug abuse counselor several times before the state facilities were used again. For those who wanted to handle their problems through local agencies (such as AA) rather than through long-term treatment (28 days) at one of the two state facilities, the counselor established an unwritten commitment that such treatment would need to be sought or some "true commitment" made if the client began to drink again.

However, once a commitment was made, the counselor was "willing to give it a shot."

A commitment was also needed by the clients to show prospective employers that their drinking problems had been addressed. Otherwise, it might be difficult to account for gaps in one's employment history or for a succession of short-term jobs. Further, the counselor would feel more comfortable as a reference for his clients when that kind of commitment had been made. When talking with prospective employers, the counselor could emphasize what clients had done and were doing to address their problems instead of having the problems overwhelm the conversation. Successful rehabilitation depended on that commitment.

Running with Cases

Perhaps more so than any other counselor, the counselor who handled the alcoholic caseload was concerned about moving cases quickly—"running with cases," as he termed it. Delay could mean lost clients, lost cases. If an individual with a drinking problem had made a commitment to address that problem, then that commitment must be supported through the agency's action. According to the counselor:

> When . . . a person who has got an alcohol problem makes a commitment for treatment, I think it is important that you move on it quickly. Even if it's not smooth, you need to get the motion going. They've made that commitment, and you need to do it. Sometimes you have to back them off a little bit. I have had people who have walked in this door, and they want to go [to a treatment facility] today. That's just not real. But, you know, they've made that commitment, and they want it right now. "Why can't I get out there this afternoon? I've decided to quit drinking." But you do try to move as fast as you can. . . . I've seen other counselors who work with alcoholics on their general caseloads don't move fast, and they come [to me] and say they lose them. I don't know how to explain that other than you need to get the motion going. You do lose a good many.

Cases were moved quickly, in both working them and concluding them. In working cases, the counselor used several strategies in "running with the cases." Applicants who were to receive long-term treatment at one of the two state facilities would often be sent there before the counselor staffed the cases at the case development staffing. The plans would be developed at the treatment facility and then amended, if necessary, by the field counselor. One casework assistant teased that such cases were "sickeningly easy." However, an applicant's high blood pressure could cause delay in arranging for the applicant to be admitted to the treatment facility. But as the counselor noted, "I'm very scared of holding people back to go to [the] treatment center unless it's . . . a dire need." To forestall such delays, the counselor would consult with his QC or with the treatment facility and let them decide whether he needed to wait or not to discuss the case with the medical consultant on her weekly visits to the office. Or, he might send the applicant to a local doctor, who would review the medical situation and write the applicant a prescription that was filled that day or the next. Once filled, the applicant was sent to the treatment facility. Because "blood pressure plays so many games with anyone," "during that withdrawal period" the counselor would ask the nursing staff of one of his referral sources to check to see if the applicant's blood pressure had stabilized once the withdrawal was completed. If not, and if "the bottom part of the blood pressure (diastolic pressure) gets above 100, then . . . we're going to see that person at least for an office visit to see if that blood pressure comes down." If at all possible, the counselor "ran with the case" to the treatment facility.

The cases of patients who were soon leaving the federal hospital were handled quickly, too. Their cases might be staffed before the counselor had obtained their hospital medical records. If the patients were to leave the hospital before the counselor returned the following week, plans might be developed at the same time as the initial interviews. The plans were typically developed the week following the initial interview, after the counselor had had a chance to review the survey and medical records. If tools or work clothes might be provided by the agency, then the counselor encouraged the patients to obtain passes to leave the hospital in order to get bids (estimates of costs from stores) on what was needed. Once the clients were discharged and working, the tools and clothes could be provided immediately.

The counselor also moved quickly when concluding cases. After his clients were successfully employed for sixty days their cases were closed. However, because the clients were claimed to be "severely disabled" due to their lengthy histories of drinking, the counselor's superiors were concerned that he was closing cases too quickly. The counselor would open a case from the federal hospital and, if all went smoothly, close it approximately two and one-half months later. The additional two weeks encompassed the opening of the case, developing the plan, waiting until the client was discharged, and job placement. As a result of his superiors' concern, the counselor and his superiors "reached a compromise" in which the counselor waited until his clients had been employed "usually at least a month" (which would "cover about the same time they would be in . . . one of . . . [the state's] treatment centers") before officially recording the start of their employment. He then followed them for the required sixty days before closing their cases. While the counselor was initially concerned that this change might adversely affect his ability to meet his goals, the change had little impact on his production. Only a few successful closures had been lost.[7]

The counselor's concern with moving quickly in serving clients led to his becoming a referral "broker" for other counselors throughout the state. Many patients at the federal hospital were returning home to cities and towns throughout the state. In the past, such patients had to endure a several-week delay as the rehabilitation counselors in their towns requested that hospital officials send the patients' records to them. Now, with the help of a casework assistant, the counselor was contacting patients who would not be staying in the local area, determining if they were interested in the agency's services, and, if so, sending photocopies of the patients' records to the area offices that would serve them. A several-week delay in moving cases was eliminated and so too were many lost cases.

Routinizing Rehabilitation Work

Rehabilitation counselors, like detectives and other human service professionals, routinize their work (Prottas, 1979: 34; Lipsky, 1980: Part III; Higgins and Butler, 1982: 129-134). Whether establishing a particular day and time for contacting referral sources, using an application form when interviewing referrals, developing and using priorities in deciding what to do next, or providing similar services to similar clients, counselors did not tackle anew each new case they began. Instead, counselors established procedures and principles that enabled them to handle different cases in similar, orderly ways. The agency's own guidelines and procedures provided an organizational routine within which counselors created their own routines. The counselor who specialized in serving those with drinking problems had routinized a great deal of his work. His two primary referral sources were routinely worked during established times on set days. His philosophy concerning the need to move cases quickly (as well as how he did so) were important parts of the routinization of his work. Most striking were the counselor's rehabilitation plans. As he noted himself, they read the same.[8]

The counselor did not claim that all alcoholics were the same. However, he felt that alcoholics faced four major problems in working successfully: sobriety, working regularly, acceptable performance, and appropriate behavior. While sobriety was the major concern, the other three problems were important, too. According to the counselor, those with drinking problems often appeared at work sporadically. When they did appear, their work performance was often inadequate, and their behavior toward others was inappropriate (for example, cussing). Therefore, the counselor focused on those four areas in the plan, in both the evaluation summary and the intermediate goals, criteria, and services. For example, in stating that the disability of alcoholism was a vocational handicap, the counselor wrote that the alcoholism

> negatively affects work performance through poor work attendance, unsatisfactory work behavior, and below average work performance.

Or that it

> negatively affects work performance through inappropriate work behavior, below standard work performance, and multiple unexcused absences.

The counselor also developed similar sets of intermediate goals, criteria, and services for his alcoholic clients. There were usually two goals, the second of which typically concerned successful employment for a minimum of sixty days. The first dealt with the four problem areas. For example:

> Maintain sobriety, work every day, perform at satisfactory work standards, and display appropriate work behavior as determined by the [federal] hospital and VR counselor through counseling and treatment.

According to the counselor, had he worked with those with diabetes, his plans would have been different, but he worked with alcoholics. However, had he in fact worked with diabetics, his plans for them would probably have been similar to each other, but in a different way than his plans for alcoholics. He and his colleagues routinized their rehabilitation work. Clients seen as similar—in terms of their disabilities, functional limitations, and perceived needs—were often served in similar ways.

CONCLUSION

As many detectives do, rehabilitation counselors and other human service professionals often specialize in their work. Through organizational and individual efforts, counselors established and worked specialty caseloads. And within the specialty caseloads, subspecialties sometimes developed. Within (and sometimes irrespective of) specializations, counselors developed procedures and philosophies that enabled them to work routinely with cases that while different, were seen to be similar in important ways. These typical features were addressed by the procedures and philosophies, each supporting the reality of the other.

As in detective details, the basic features of rehabilitation work are displayed in the specialty caseloads, though the specifics and their significance may vary. For example, establishing and working referral sources were important to the counselors who handled the hearing-impaired, school, and alcoholic caseloads. Concluding cases was the primary task of the public offender counselor. In order to make a case, school counselors needed to sell their agency to the referrals. The counselor who handled the alcoholic caseload "ran with" cases in order to move them quickly. And tangibles were a concern to all, particularly to public offender counselors, who sweetened their agency's offerings with "sugar money" but sometimes found the taste bitter. The basic features of rehabilitation work are grounded in the specifics of specialty caseloads, and those specifics display the variety in rehabilitation work.

While detectives see their job as catching "real" criminals and clearing cases, in doing so, they aim to serve justice. Rehabilitation counselors, like other human service professionals, work and conclude cases and manage caseloads. They do so in order to serve those in need. Concern has been growing as to how well justice is served by detectives (and the criminal justice system of which they are a part) and about how just (as well as effective, efficient, and so forth) the service of human service professionals and agencies is (Lipsky, 1980; Reiman, 1984). Perhaps the growing concerns about justice and service are not all that different. If justice is not always served, then perhaps service is not always just. If not, then why not and what can be done? In response to those two questions, I conclude my investigation.

NOTES

1. For example, how counselors use their time in various activities, such as counseling, placement, and intake, varies by the type of caseload (Wright, 1980: 173).

2. I would have liked to observe the mental health caseload closely, but I was not able to make arrangements to do so. One counselor who handled the caseload believed that I would "get in the way." The "workers compensation" caseload was a small one in which much of the counselor's responsiblity invovled screening such cases on file with the Industrial Commission to determine which should be referred to counselors throughout the state.

3. A GAO (1982: 6-7) audit criticized agencies' practices of providing physical restoration services to clients who often did not possess substantial handicaps to employment. The audit cited the following case:

> A 56-year-old [state] client diagnosed as having a hearing impairment was claimed as a successful rehabilitation after the rehabilitation agency paid $37 to repair the person's hearing aid. At the time of the referral, the client was working as a border guard earning $633 per month and remained in this job after the rehabilitation services were provided.

The counselor's and the agency's emphasis on substantial services was in part a response to avoid such criticism.

4. See Colvin (1972) for a brief history and overview of vocational rehabilitation of the public offender.

5. Based on figures supplied by a counselor who disagreed that the public offender caseload was a relatively quick-turnover one, the average time recently from referral to successful closure for public offender cases was approximately twelve months, compared to twenty for the entire agency's cases. Further, because the cases were opened while the offenders were in prison, the field counselors had responsibility for the cases only part of the time they were open.

6. One counselor who did not handle public offenders recounted an incident in which the client of a public offender counselor came to the area office for a maintenance check. The counselor was absent, and a supervisory person was simply planning to give the client his check. Instead, the counselor who told me the story learned the client was working, where he was working, and other pertinent information before the client left with his maintenance check.

7. The counselor also "walked" with cases, too. If he did not feel the applicants/clients had made a commitment to deal with their drinking, or if some kind of training were involved, the counselor went more slowly. Other counselors in the state who handled alcoholic caseloads did not necessarily "run with their cases." According to the local counselor, one such colleague interviewed clients several times before arranging for treatment at one of the state's facilities. Certainly different "styles" emerge within rehabilitation work.

8. Some have argued that such routinization, often involving stereotypes, limits human service professionals in serving clients (Salomone, 1970: 15; Lipsky, 1976: 207-208). Certainly it may. Yet without routinization, could human service professionals serve clients at all?

7

CONCLUSION
Redoing Human Service Work

Detectives work cases and make investigations in order to deal with "righteous crime" and "real criminals" (Sanders, 1977: 80). Their job is to catch criminals and clear cases. In doing so, they seek to serve justice. However, concern continues as to how well justice is served by detectives and, more generally, by the criminal justice system of which they are a part. One has only to open the newspaper or a news magazine or turn on the television almost any day to be confronted with concerns about the criminal justice system. While the concerns vary greatly depending on the perspectives of the critics, they include the following: coddling criminals, official corruption, entrapment, plea bargaining, a hamstrung criminal justice system, inadequate resources, a "lock-them-up" mentality, too lenient punishment, too harsh punishment, discrimination, assembly-line justice, and even no justice. Perhaps the harshest indictment is that the criminal justice system is criminal, not just:

> The criminal justice system in America is morally indistinguishable from criminality because it exercises force and imposes suffering on human beings *while violating its own morally justifying ideals: protection and justice* [Reiman, 1984: 153].

Rehabilitation counselors and other human service professionals work and conclude cases and manage caseloads. They do so in order to serve those "in need." Yet, just as concern has been growing regarding how well justice is served by detectives and the criminal justice system of which they are a part, so too has concern been growing regarding how just (and effective, efficient, humane, and so forth) is the service of human service professionals and the agencies of which they are a part. Are human service agencies increasingly becoming "crazy systems," which are both inscrutable and unaccountable (Singer, 1980)? Might those most in need receive the least and those least in need receive the most (Rein, 1980: 87)? Might services not be *merely* ineffective but also hazardous to the life and well-being of those who receive them (McKinlay, 1978)? One observer concludes that the

> end result of the depressing collage of thousands of fragmented and depersonalized services, offered by a disenchanted and alienated staff to frustrated and confused poor consumers, is the moral, social, and fiscal bankruptcy of sizable segments of our society [Huber, 1977: 27].

Rather than enabling, the human service professions many have become partially disabling (Illich et al., 1977).

Human service work is increasingly recognized as problematic. It seems beset by shortcomings of imagination, intention, and implementation. My aim here is not to explore all those shortcomings—look to others for that.[1] My aim is much more modest. Rather, given the metaphor of detective work, which has enlightened my investigation of rehabilitation counselors and other human service professionals, what can be said about the shortcomings in doing human service work? And once those shortcomings have been identified, how might we think about addressing them?

SHORTCOMINGS IN SERVICE

Throughout my investigation of rehabilitation and other human service professionals, I have stressed that human service work occurs within an organization, set within a conflictual society, and composed of policies, procedures, and other professionals. To understand the shortcomings in service, we need to look again at the social circumstances in which service is provided (Lipsky, 1980: Part IV). Of course, the same is true for detective work. The "defects" of detective (and criminal justice) work are paralleled by the "disabilities" of rehabilitation (and other human service work).

Defects of Detective Work

Detectives, like all human service professionals, work within organizations that are "embodiments of contradictory tendencies in American society as a whole" (Lipsky, 1980: 1983). The goals of the organization may be "unclear or contradictory because they reflect the contradictory impulses of the society the agency serves" (Lipsky, 1980: 165). Within the contradictions of society toward crime and law enforcement, detectives and others within the criminal justice system do their work. It is no wonder, then, that such work should be problematic. What an English barrister said of the (British) police applies well to detectives and others who do criminal justice work:

> The public use the police as a scapegoat for its neurotic attitude toward crime. Janus-like we have always turned two faces toward a policeman. We employ him to administer the law, and yet ask him to waive it. We resent him when he enforces the law in our own case, yet demand his dismissal when he does not elsewhere. We offer him bribes, yet denounce his corruption. We expect him to be a member of society, yet not to share its values. We admire violence, even against society itself, but condemn force by the police in our behalf. We tell the police that they are entitled to information from the public, yet we ostracize informers. We ask for crime to be eradicated, but only by use of "sporting" methods [cited in Morris and Hawkins, 1970: 89-90].

To the extent that American society continues to hold contradictory expectations for detectives and others who work in the criminal justice system, their work is likely to be problematic.

Detective work arises out of the organization in which the work is done. If detectives work within an organization were "stats"—arrest and clearance statistics—have great significance, then detectives will do their work in such a way that they produce those stats (Skolnick, 1966; Waegel, 1981). In producing stats, they may engage in *routine* practices that others find problematic. In order to produce a "steady stream of arrests," detectives may "skim" cases. By "selectively working only those cases which appear potentially solvable from information contained in the original report," and "summarily suspending the remainder of ordinary cases," detectives produce arrests (Waegel, 1981: 267). However, while supervisors are aware of such practices, their performance may be assessed by superiors in "crude quantitative terms." A decrease in arrests becomes a cause for concern. Consequently, "supervisors support the practices of skimming even though they recognize that it ensures that a majority of ordinary cases will never receive a thorough investigation" (Waegel, 1981: 267-268). Problematic practices are often a response to the problems posed by the organization.

Detectives are being equally pragmatic when they swap reduced charges for suspects' confessions to solve previously unsolved crimes (Skolnick, 1966: 167-181). Justice may suffer, but crimes have been cleared. Looking good has become doing good, but only because we do not take the trouble to look closely. We become satisfied with the pronouncements of our law enforcement officials, and then, because we hold them to the logic of their pronouncements (that is, arrests/clearances equal justice), they become "caught" in their own "trap."

Yet even where the organization seeks to deal with "righteous crime" and "real criminals," with "big" cases, detectives will also give some cases little investigative attention. "Little" cases typically receive "little" attention (Sanders, 1977: 95-96). And the same strategy by detectives in narcotics and vice, who typically rely on informants in order to know about crime, may lead to questionable practices. Informants' offenses may be overlooked, while money and other desirables (such as reduced charges) are exchanged for their cooperation. Perhaps justice is served and denied through such practices (Skolnick, 1966: chaps. 6, 7; Gilsinan, 1982: 57-58). Many of the "excesses" (such as entrapment) of detectives may be best understood as the practical, often routine, responses of ordinary people to the demands of the organization in which they work.

The nature of detective work leads to problematic practices, too. While we often think law enforcement officials are the "first line of defense" against crime, in reality, citizens are the first to respond. Much of law enforcement, as noted earlier, is reactive. Police and detectives react to the complaints of citizens. To do otherwise often would prove much too intrusive for a democratic society. (Of course, when law enforcement does otherwise, such as in undercover work that may lead to provocation and entrapment, some citizens become concerned.) Thus, in order to do their jobs, detectives must depend greatly on the cooperation of citizens—victims and witnesses. To the extent that such cooperation is problematic, and it often is (witness victims' low rate of notifying law enforcement officials; U.S. Department of Justice, 1981), detective work is likely to be problematic, too.[2]

Concerned with the task of solving *many* puzzles (typically too many to solve), in which all the pieces to each puzzle are not known beforehand, detective work is inherently problematic. Set that task within organizational and societal concerns, and there is little wonder that detectives develop, use, and explain their behavior through the use of routine practices, procedures, and philosophies. While detective work is an ongoing accomplishment (Sanders, 1977: 129), it is accomplished through the use of and reference to routine practices and understandings. Events that are unique become kinds of cases that are similar or different, some to be investigated and others to be disposed of quickly. Of course, those familiar with the criminal justice system recognize well that such routine handling of crime is the system's routine (Sudnow, 1965; Gilsinan, 1982; Higgins and Butler, 1982: 129-134). Uniformity and comparability, which we presumably want when justice is done, can be overdone through typification and routinization. Yet some of it must be done if detective work is to be accomplished. The "defects" of detective work are not simply due to deficiencies in detectives, but to the contradictions and complexities of the social circumstances in which the work is done. So it is for the work of rehabilitation counselors and other human service professionals as well.

Disabilities of Rehabilitation

Federal audits of vocational rehabilitation throughout the country, to which I have referred throughout the book, have uncovered practices of rehabilitation professionals some consider questionable. Of course, many of these (functionally limiting) practices have been addressed by the agencies. Some of them were (still are?) as follows:

About $1,290 was paid for training a student for 33 weeks to be a counter helper at a restaurant. The student had already worked at this position for 10 months [GAO, 1977: 11].

A 19-year-old [state] client with mental retardation[IQ, 75] was claimed as a successful rehabilitation after the agency provided a pair of work shoes and a general medical examination at a total cost of $52. The vocational plan of material handler was written several days after the client began work in the same factory that employed his father [GAO, 1982: 13].

A 17-year-old [state] client with an allergy condition was provided $158 for treatment for this problem and $3,040 to attend music training at a State university. The client quit school without notifying the counselors; consequently, there was a 16-month loss of contract. The counselor found out from the client's sister that the client had quit school and gone to work as a music store sales person. The [state] agency closed this case as a successful rehabilitation [GAO, 1982: 8].

It is too simple and not particularly enlightening to claim that these "disabilities" of rehabilitation are due to the offensive actions of unprofessional rehabilitation professionals. Instead, just as many of the "defects" of detective work are best seen as practical, often officially sanctioned, responses to the demands (organizational, societal, and inherent in the activity) detectives confront, so too are the "disabling" practices of rehabilitation professionals (and other human service workers) best understood as practical, often accepted, responses to the demands they face.

If society has pitied, scorned, and then belatedly and "charitably" (though sometimes begrudingly) extended a hand to aid the disabled, then organizations mandated to serve them are unlikely to have clear missions (Bowe, 1978). If worth is achieved through work, but dignity inheres in being human, then vocational rehabilitation agencies may be caught between jobs and justice. Vocational rehabilitation, like other human services, is provided by a society often confused and contradictory in its concerns and commitments. No wonder some of the practices of rehabilitation may be "disabling."

If within rehabilitation organizations "stats"—status 26 closures—are important, then counselors are likely to do their work to produce "stats." The number of clients successfully rehabilitated by counselors is strongly related to the goals set by their agencies (Zadny and James, 1979a). However, some of their practices may appear questionable, at least to those who are not subject to the goals. When counselors develop and work referral sources likely to produce "good" referrals (even if that means accepting some "bad" ones), manage contacts with referrals so those who may be inappropriate screen themselves out, do not take applications on all who are referred, move cases quickly, use "sugar money" and other tangibles to create and maintain clients' interest and cooperation, catch clients working, "treat the record," and engage in many other practices explored in the previous pages, they are responding to the demands and circumstances they encounter. From this perspective, they are competently and often with great ingenuity doing rehabilitation work, work expected of them by their organizational superiors and assented to by us.

A great deal of rehabilitation and other human service work involves working with many, often too many, people, given the available resources (Lipsky, 1980: 33-39). In managing caseloads, counselors not only parcel out limited time, energy, and resources among many in need, but they also sometimes "benignly neglect" the need of some in order to serve others. For example, if counselors jeopardized their reputations with employers by sending them questionable clients who want to work but fail in doing so, then they may have difficulty rehabilitating others. When counselors put uncooperative clients on hold so that they can more efficiently and often effectively spend their time and energy on others, they are being "practical." Their practices reflect that they recognize the demands of working with many cases. However, the "questionable" client and the uncooperative client may in fact have the greatest need of a counselor's attention. Risks must be taken and time and energy spent if these clients are to be served. Yet, through service that may ultimately not prove enabling to some, others will go unserved. Rehabilitation counselors did not develop this dilemma, but they must respond to it.

Like detectives, rehabilitation counselors and other human service professionals often confront many puzzling situations—that is the nature of their work. Yet, if the situations were to remain puzzling, obviously they would get little work done. So they (and their agencies) routinize their work. They develop and use classification schemes, standard practices, common understandings, and other means of serving people who are unique, but who, in important ways, become served as if they were similar. Could it be otherwise? Perhaps to a degree (which is important), but not likely in kind (Lipsky, 1980: 84-85, 199). Therefore, when it is claimed that "all (clients) must be served on an individual basis, that is, there must be a unique plan for service based upon the unique needs and resources of each applicant" (Wright, 1980: 169), or when we are warned that "assurances [of individuality in human service] should not be so easily taken for granted" (Murphy and Ursprung, 1983: 12), both the claim and the warning reflect an idealized, but certainly mistaken, view of human service work. While routinization may often be overdone, it is only through routinization that human service work gets done at all.

Finally, rehabilitation counselors and other human service professionals, like detectives, do their work with and for others. Perhaps this point is so obvious that its significance is often overlooked. Clients are not merely served by professionals, but through their active participation they serve themselves (Gartner, 1977: 2). However, that participation is often problematic. The understandings and interests of those to be served may or may not be particularly compatible with the understandings and interests of the service professionals and their agencies. Of course, as we know, the "true" professional works "out" and works "through" those differences. How idealistic—and condescending! Such a view assumes an omnipotence among professionals that is not realized among mere mortals. It disregards the will of clients; it assumes that clients can be "bent" (often camouflaged as "counseled," "instructed," or "shown") to what the professionals and the agencies know is best for them. In candid and reflective moments, human service professionals realize they often do not know what is best for themselves, let alone others, and that even the most seemingly compliant client can become at odds with the (intended) course of services. Yet, if the dependency of disability (and poverty, ignorance, and so on) is to be "truly" undone, is compliance even called for (DeJong, 1983)? From the demands faced by human services professionals come the shortcomings of service.

"REHABILITATING" REHABILITATION

If we need to help the criminal justice system "go straight," as one critic has argued (Reiman, 1984: 153), then perhaps rehabilitation and other human service agencies need to be "rehabilitated." Just as I did not pursue all the "disabilities" of rehabilitation, I do not intend to offer a detailed, point-by-point program (the goals, criteria, and services) for rehabilitating rehabilitation. Instead, based on the metaphor of detective work, I will suggest what should not be seen as a panacea for rehabilitation and other human service agencies. I will also propose some general principles regarding what might be done to "rehabilitate" rehabilitation and the problems likely to occur if those steps are taken.

Unlikely Panaceas

A common set of suggestions for improving human service work, which is voiced now particularly in reference to education, seems to rest on an assumption similar to a long-standing (though fluctuating) assumption concerning criminal justice personnel. The assumption, stated crudely, is that cops are as "crooked" as criminals. From that assumption flow several strategies for improving criminal justice work, strategies also called for to improve human service work. The strategies aim to improve the competence and conduct of human service professionals. First, recruit and develop "better" professionals through "improved" training and selection. If we believe that human services can enhance those who receive it, then it makes sense to suggest that improved selection and training of human service professionals will enhance their abilities to serve others. Thus, with understandable pride, human service administrators point to the advanced degrees and certifications of their professionals and the on-the-job training they receive. Second, and somewhat inconsistent with the first strategy, administrators need to supervise more effectively (that is, control) the service providers. Hence supervisors, quality control specialists, forms, paperwork, audits, internal investigation units, and other means for checking on the service providers proliferate. In vocational rehabilitation, programs may already be "close to control saturation in the form of supervision and procedural requirements imposed on the service delivery personnel." One individual performing supervision for "every 2.5 direct service workers" in some agencies would strike many of us as saturation (Crisler et al., 1980: 53).

While better training and increased supervision may do no harm and may do some good (certainly "basic" levels of individual competence need to be assured if they can be decided upon), such strategies individualize shortcomings that are social and organizational, not personal, in nature. Given the tremendous growth of regulations, evaluations, reports, audits, supervision, and the like, human service work remains problematic. While more may at times be better, after a point it may be useless or worse (Prottas, 1979: Part IV; but see Hasenfeld, 1980). Any familiarity with the problems that beset the "true" professions, such as law and medicine, in which presumably the practitioners are highly trained, selected, and motivated, indicates that more professional professionals will not be the panacea for human service work (Lipsky, 1980: 201-204).

Substantial Responses

If the problems of rehabilitation and other human service work arise from social circumstances (the contradictions of society and the demands of the organization), then "tinkering" with the providers may be more manageable for and less threatening to society and its service organizations, but it may be less effective, too.[3] Perhaps the sources of the problems, not the symptoms, should be addressed. While this would be difficult to do, the results may be more meaningful (Lipsky, 1980: Part IV). I have several suggestions that follow from the analogy to detective work.

Rehabilitation counselors, like detectives, produce, to a great extent, what is expected of them. If both are expected to produce "numbers," then detectives produce arrests and counselors produce 26s. If rehabilitation counselors (and other human service professionals) are expected to produce quality, to really serve those in need, as they have been increasingly expected to do, then they are indeed likely do so (Zadny and James, 1979a; see Chapter 2, also). While it may be useful to propose and evaluate techniques and strategies for producing quality, I suspect that counselors will develop practices for doing so, much as they have for producing quantity. Let the counselors share their procedures with their colleagues and supervisors (Lipsky, 1980: 200-201, 206-207).[4] After all, through training and selection, more competent and concerned professionals are working in human service agencies.

Such a change requires that organizations (and society) do not put the professionals in a bind: expecting them to achieve quantity and quality, often in the face of diminishing resources and rising demands. This was a bind some counselors in the rehabilitation agency I observed noted, as the new policy that cut bill paying in favor of substantial services went into effect. Of course, here is where a difficulty emerges. How many people can professionals serve "well"? Because there is no easy response to that question, to assume there is (as reflected in the attitude that it is a technical matter of calculating goals for the year) leads to more difficulties than are necessary.

A caution: Except for outright falsification (which I suspect is rare), the routine practices developed by rehabilitation professionals to achieve what they traditionally have been directed to achieve—quantity—have to a great degree been organizationally accepted. Outsiders not confronting the demands of the organization have criticized some of those practices. Given a new direction to ensure quality, counselors are likely to develop new practices and modify present ones to do so. Thus they are likely to engage in practices that will be criticized by outsiders who do not face the (new) demands and constraints encountered by the counselors. For example, as there has been a greater emphasis on serving the severely disabled, I am sure (though I did not investigate this carefully) there has been an increase in the practice of classifying as severely disabled clients who previously had not been labeled as such. Does that mean the clients are not severely disabled and only through the stroke of a pen have become so? No. Some of the classifications will be accepted by outsiders, others will not. Responding to different demands (such as the agency's demand to have a high percentage of successfully closed clients who are severely disabled or that of the GAO to be the government's watchdog), the critics and the criticized may disagree about the propriety of those and other practices. Fair enough. But to conclude quickly that the criticized are at fault is merely finger-pointing. A proliferation of rules may redefine how counselors are to define clients, but judgments will always be made. Isn't that what professionals are supposed to do? To the extent that the rules (and the reviews) do proliferate, the "human" may be taken out of human service work.

If rehabilitation counselors and other human service professionals can be understood as detectives, then at least two more substantive responses follow. First, while police and detectives do act as judge and jury (we both expect them to do so and criticize them for doing so), there are separate bodies of judges and juries (and attorneys) to review, even to contest, what police and detectives do. Might that principle, if certainly not the practice (and the problems that have accompanied it), be applied to human service professionals? The need for information that represents and assesses the experiences of those involved in human service organizations and that is collected and analyzed independent of such organizations is recognized (Nagi, 1974). Why not go further? To an extent, such steps have taken through appeal mechanisms, ombudsmen, and community advocates (Nagi, 1974). While many human service clients are voluntary (and in that respect different from criminal offenders), all are not. And to the extent that typically there are few alternatives, voluntary clients become more like involuntary clients if they continue to want services. Should the human service agencies that make and conclude cases also pass judgment on them, on their making and conclusion? Perhaps not. This does not mean that human service professionals cannot be or are not fair. They can and they are. Instead, this suggestion recognizes that human service work is as complex, problematic, and filled with the differing concerns of the participants as the work of detectives and the criminal justice system. We do not rely solely on the good intentions of detectives and the police (though maybe we should not so easily suspect their intentions). Perhaps we should not do so for human service professionals (and their agencies either). No adversary system is envisioned, but through some form of representation the client's concerns may be championed more effectively.

Second, and related to the first response, the "clients" of criminal justice agencies, the victims and offenders, are eminently more knowledgeable about their situations and the agencies designed to serve them than are those who might be served by rehabilitation and many other human service agencies. Citizens have much better knowledge of crime and criminal justice agencies than they have of disabilities and rehabilitation agencies (see Chapter 5), though, typically, citizens are dangerously ignorant of all the agencies that serve them (Lipsky, 1980: 53). Society and the criminal justice system take for granted that victims know when they need to be served (though they may not ask to be served) and now take for granted that, through independent representation, the accused have become (more) competent advocates for their interests.[5] Citizens, particularly those who, by circumstance or condition, are not highly competent advocates for their interests, must have the opportunity to develop that competency (independent of the agencies that serve them; Gartner et al., 1979).[6] If those served are in part the producers of the service, then perhaps it makes sense for them to be as knowledgeable as possible when they seek service, rather than *after* they have been served. To the extent that citizens have the knowledge and capacity to make reasoned decisions on their own, they will be better served and better able to serve themselves (DeJong, 1983).

For example, relatively few people referred to vocational rehabilitation agencies know much, if anything, about the agencies. If they were more knowledgeable about the agencies, their procedures and services, they could pursue their interests more effectively (see Chapter 3). They would also be more likely to seek services than (possibly) be referred by others. Instead, they depend greatly on professionals for whom clients' interests are only one concern to which they must respond and to which they respond differentially.

If rehabilitation and other human service work is to be enabling rather than possibly disabling, then the dependency of disability (and poverty, ignorance, and the like) must be undone. But that will be difficult because through human services agencies "society organizes the control, restriction, and maintenance of relatively powerless groups" (Lipsky, 1980: 191). To "rehabilitate" rehabilitation and other human service agencies, we need to "rehabilitate" ourselves.[7]

CONCLUSION

Rehabilitation counselors, mental health professionals, parole agents, and other human service professionals do detective work. And doing detective work, whether it be law enforcement or human service, is often problematic. Justice may not be served and service may not be just. However, to individualize the shortcomings of service is to make scapegoats out of ordinary people. To do so fails to recognize that the work of human service professionals (and the shortcomings of that work) arise from the social circumstances, from the contradictions of society and the demands of the service agencies, in which the work is done. Therefore, just as rehabilitation counselors and other human service professions aim to place responsibility for failure where they believe it belongs—often on the clients (Lipsky, 1976: 205)—so I want to place responsibility for any shortcomings of service where I believe it belongs—on us. To the extent that our increasingly service-oriented society is "defined by the quality of life as measured by [its] services and amenities" (Bell, 1972: 166), our character is tested by our response to the shortcomings of those services.

NOTES

1. See the following for further discussion of the problems of human services and human service work (Illich, 1971, 1975; Hasenfeld and English, 1974: Lipsky, 1976, 1980; Bogdan and Biklen, 1977; Prottas, 1979). An indictment of human service work follows that is as harsh as that mentioned of the criminal justice system:

> My concern here can be put quite simply: How ethical is it for one group of people (possibly overrepresenting the middle classes) to deliver to another group (primarily those with social needs) services which are largely ineffective and increasingly hazardous but which are supported to an ever-increasing extent by the state? It may be that one latent consequence of our well-intentioned desire to achieve full employment through the perpetual expansion of the human service sector will be to further institutionalize inequality—albeit in the name of altruism and service. In other words, liberal policy makers, in advocating the expansion of human services, may be fostering a state of affairs which results in the rigidification of a system that is the converse of that which they are striving to achieve [McKinlay, 1978: 34].

2. The use and abuse of informants are partially an outgrowth of the conflict concerning cooperation.

3. However, focusing criticism on the professionals, criticism often directed their way by citizens, does serve to deflect attention from organizational and societal concerns and practices that give rise to the criticized behavior of the professionals (Lipsky, 1980: 184).

4. However, quality of performance and—more important, I think—of outcome (though the two are often interwined) may be difficult to measure and may be likely to conflict with the emphasis on minimizing costs and increasing productivity (Lipsky, 1980: 168-172). Of course, the conflict points to the contradictions of society in which service agencies work to serve society.

5. Of course, what is taken for granted perhaps should not be, not because it is faulty, but, in being so obvious, its realization may not be carefully and continually provided for in practice.

6. For several reasons it may be problematic to service providers to be advocates for those they serve. In general, being an advocate is "incompatible with their [human service professionals'] need to judge and control clients for bureaucratic purposes" (Lipsky, 1980: 73).

7. "For just as I believe that America handicaps disabled people, and by doing so handicaps itself as well, so too do I believe that America can rehabilitate not only its citizens who are disabled but itself as well" (Bowe, 1980: xiv).

RESEARCH APPENDIX
The Sociological Detective

If the work of rehabilitation counselors and other human service professionals can be understood usefully through the metaphor of detective work, then perhaps so can the research of sociologists. Both detectives and sociologists are interested in determining what happened, why it happened, and when it will happen again. In doing so, detectives attempt to solve crimes and sociologists attempt to develop understanding of social behavior. When doing so, there are likely to be some differences in the methods used. For example, detectives rely more heavily on physical evidence than do sociologists, while sociologists might employ sophisticated statistical analyses (Sanders, 1976: 1-2). However, there is an important difference between detective and sociological work about which many social scientists are unlikely to agree. It is an important difference, however, to me.

To those who confront the work of detectives, how the detectives have done their work is often as important as what they have done. Procedures are important. What detectives have accomplished (as well as their competence/ morality) may be called into question by the questionable methods of their accomplishments. One example of this is that damming evidence may be disallowed if it was gathered illegally. Of course, techniques are important in detective work of all kinds. The findings are often judged by the techniques used to achieve them. Suspect techniques cast suspicion on the findings. Isn't some of the concern about human service work actually about the techniques used by the workers? This stance characterizes sociological and other scientific investigations. "If research is done by the correct, proper formula or method, then the results are adequate, valid, correct. (If not, then they are not.) That is the common view," but it is not the only view (Stewart and Tucker, 1983: 1).

In what follows, I will briefly discuss my investigation of the work of rehabilitation counselors. Like other field researchers, I will detail the number of interviews conducted, the number of pages of notes accumulated, and the like. I will explain how I did the research and describe important issues that emerged in the process. I will modestly mention the limitations of the research while implicitly suggesting the strength of the results. All this is said to impress others and to convince them that the researchers know about what they are writing (Johnson, 1975: 186). Do not be taken in. If after reading this work you can better address whatever you are confronting, then this work has merit for you. Merit does not reside in the scholarliness of the work. It exists through its use and, therefore, varies by its uses (or lack thereof). Techniques may help researchers produce works that have merit to others, but that merit cannot be judged by the adequacy of the techniques. Does that mean that anything goes in research? No. Lying, coercion, and other improprieties are committed by sociological detectives (as well as other kinds of detectives). Such improprieties should be place within the social context of "doing research," not merely seen as the result of the personal shortcomings of social scientists. Such improprieties may lead to findings that have merit to others. However, merit cannot justify all means.

In discussing my sociological investigation of rehabilitation counselors, I first present "just the facts"—what was done in conducting the research. After doing so, I discuss the elements of the investigation, important concerns that emerged from the research (and, in part, how they were addressed). Finally, I mention some "reasonable doubts" of the case, some limitations of the research.

JUST THE FACTS

After preliminary contact and discussion with rehabilitation professionals in late 1978 and early 1979, I began the sociological investigation in the spring of 1979. Throughout the spring and summer, I primarily interviewed the professional staff of the local area office I was observing and went to a few meetings. As I began work on two other books (Higgins, 1980; Higgins and Butler, 1982), my investigation of rehabilitation counselors (which now included some observations of their work in the field) became less frequent in fall 1979 and was then put on hold until late 1980. After some (re) contacts with local area office and state-level professionals, I began my research again (perhaps "began again" states the case more accurately than does "continue") in the spring of 1981. I gathered the bulk of my field information from spring 1981 through summer 1982. Follow-up interviews in fall 1982 and then much later, in summer 1983, were conducted. Analysis, and then writing, rewriting, and additional analysis occurred primarily from late summer 1982 through fall 1984. A rough draft of this work was then shown to the rehabilitation professionals. Their comments and those from fellow social scientists were used in rewriting the book.

As I noted in Chapter 2, I investigated a local area office situated in a metroplitan region of a state that was widely recognized as a leader in vocational rehabilitation. Due to the protection of the professionals' and the agency's identities, I will say no more about where the research was conducted. Later I will note some limitations that possibly arose out of the research being concluded in one area office of one agency.

During the major period of my investigation, I interviewed and/or expressly observed the activities of more than 90 percent (approximately 30) of the counselors, supervisory personnel, and consultants who worked out of the two main offices or the school projects in the local area office I observed.[1] I also observed the activities of several counselors in the case development staffings and/or case manual study group who did not want to participate "directly" in my investigation. Including the initial phase and the major period of the research, I interviewed and/or expressly observed approximately 40 members of the rehabilitation staff.

By interviewing professional staff, accompanying them during their work, observing staff meetings, case development staffing, and consultations, and examining the case manual and counselors' case folders, I accumulated more than 3000 pages of double-spaced, typed notes. Approximately one-third of the notes were transcriptions of taped interviews, one-third were notes of observations of counselors' activities, and one-third were of case development staffings. I observed approximately 100 case development staffings and tape-recorded them soon after I began attending them (the end of March 1981) until mid-May. My remaining notes on observations of CDSs (throughout 1981 and then less frequently until spring 1982, with a few follow-ups in June 1982) were handwritten. When accompanying counselors in and out of the office, I wrote notes both in and out of their presence (for example, when they left their offices to talk with their assistants), though they always knew I was or would be taking notes.

THE ELEMENTS OF THE INVESTIGATION

In doing field research, issues often emerge, such as access to those who are to be understood, their trust and cooperation, and the impact the researcher has on those observed (Johnson, 1975). Researchers must also be concerned that they do not mistake the unusual for the ordinary. Finally, how do researchers develop a framework to organize their observations and thoughts in order to tell a sociological story?

In gaining and later regaining access to the rehabilitation organization, I met with local and state supervisory personnel and with the area office professional staff. At the time, I explained my research as an investigation of "complex decision making in a service organization." Supervisory personnel were interested in what I might learn and share with them. They were concerned, however, that I not be merely trying to find fault with their organization. I told them and others repeatedly that I did not intend to judge them, that I would share my ideas with them before they were published, that their identities would not be revealed, and that I was simply interested in understanding what counselors were doing. If they felt it was necessary, then they could make whatever changes in procedures they deemed appropriate. Given the refusal/reluctance of two other human services agencies I approached before and during this project, the willingness of the rehabilitation agency and its staff to let an outsider come in was greatly appreciated.

Trust and cooperation can be fragile, perhaps never fully realized, and often changing. I am not sure how researchers (or people in any situation) develop the trust and cooperation of those they seek to understand.[2] I am not sure how a researcher knows how much trust and cooperation have been extended by those being observed. By sharing with the rehabilitation professionals what I was doing and why and by being interested enough to understand their concerns and not judge their actions, I believe a "workable" level of trust and cooperation was extended to me. However, several professionals were not interested in being involved in my investigation, and two other professionals' trust and cooperation fluctuated throughout the investigation. At times they did not want me to accompany and/or interview them, but later they allowed me to do so. By being accommodating to their wishes and unassuming, I was reextended their help, which became substantial. At the CDS meetings and throughout my investigation, counselors had more to concern themselves with than my presence. Infrequently they "played" to the tape recorder I used for a while at CDS meetings. They noted to colleagues that it was on, and, therefore, one needed to be careful what one said (this occurred only a few times), or they mentioned they had been a little nervous before I interviewed them. Counselors remarked that I did not disrupt their encounters with referrals, applicants, and clients (though sometimes I was not allowed to sit with a counselor who was counseling a particular client, such as one with a psychological disability who might be nervous due to my presence). That counselors in my presence talked and acted in ways that could have led to their being sanctioned is probably an indication that certainly some trust and cooperation were extended to me.

However, trust and cooperation develop out of a situation to which the researcher comes but over which he or she has previously had no control (Johnson, 1975: 73). Several professional staff noted that audits of the agency before my arrival probably made it more difficult for me. The researcher's wider contacts in the community may also disrupt the investigation. My wife teaches deaf children and I know many of the professional staff involved in educating those children in the local school district. After having accompanied one counselor into a high school program for hearing-impaired children, school officials expressed some concern about my presence. For a short time it seemed that, the permission given to me to accompany the counselors into the field, might be rescinded. Researchers must work continually at encouraging the trust and cooperation of those they seek to understand, but they need to be prepared for that trust and cooperation to fluctuate, sometimes dramatically.

Certainly my presence had no major impact on the rehabilitation work. While the reactivity of researchers is a real concern, it is probably a much greater concern to researchers than to those being observed. As I previously noted, counselors had more important concerns than to worry about me. My presence at CDS was unremarkable, though the counselors did wonder where I was when I missed two meetings in a row at the time of my daughter's birth. According to the counselors, I seemed to have little adverse impact on the referrals, applicants, and clients. I was just Mr. Higgins or Professor Higgins from the university, who was accompanying the counselor today. (No client objected to my presence.) However, in smaller ways, I did have some impact on counselor's rehabilitation work.

Several times I provided job leads, one of which I know was successful. I helped locate clients' homes when I accompanied counselors on their home visits, and several female counselors said they were glad that I had accompanied them. Several times counselors asked me what I thought about a client or about a client's situation. Once, I mentioned to a counselor that I believed one of his clients would be likely to become upset if his tuition support to a technical college was cut off, because it did not seem that the client realized such could happen if he did not maintain a "C" average. At times clients talked with me when the counselor was interrupted by a phone call or left the office. I always felt uncomfortable when that happened because I did not want to influence the client, particularly if I had not been asked by the counselor for my suggestions. Counselors infrequently reworded their R-1 notes after I had asked them to read the notes to me. They did so because when they reread the notes they interpreted the original statement as perhaps incomplete or misleading. For example, one time a counselor noted that a client did not appear at his home, although the counselor waited one hour. Upon reflection, the counselor realized that such documentation made it seem as if the client had not kept an appointment, when actually he did not know about the recent developments in his case (a physical was needed so the client could begin work in a few days). Therefore, the counselor reworded the R-1 notes. Finally, at times counselors shared with me their personal concerns and difficulties. By offering supportive responses, I trust that I did not exacerbate their concerns or troubles.

In attempting to understand human service professionals and others, a danger emerges that researchers will mistake the exceptional for the routine, the highly problematic for the ordinary. For instance, in a study of a group medical practice, the physicians

did not talk to each other or to the interviewers about their routines. They talked about their crises. They did not talk about slow days, but about those days when the work pressure seemed overhelming. . . . It was by the problematic that they symbolized their work, and it was in terms of the problematic, even when it constituted a small proportion of their work, that they evaluated their practices [Freidson, 1975: 48].

Consequently, researchers need to be careful in evaluating what is told to them (Roth, 1972: 850-851).

I faced that potential pitfall. Frequently the CDS involved discussion of problematic cases. By understanding what is problematic, a researcher can also understand what is routine. Certainly CDS was often recognized by counselors as routine. At other times counselors apologized for "boring" me because so little action took place when I sat in their offices during part of the day. Or they told me they wanted to make sure that they had a full schedule so I would not be bored. Being bored did not bother me (rarely was I) because I realized that most human service work, even that typically seen as exciting or dangerous, such as police work or medical work, is usally mundane and routine.

If sociologists sometimes tell stories, then where do their plots, their frameworks, come from? When I began my investigation of rehabilitation counselors, I did not have in mind the metaphor of detective work. In the fall of 1981 I was tentatively using the framework of "rehabilitating the deserving" in order to get a handle on what I was learning. Through federal and state policy and through the actions of the counselors and other staff, some people were designated as appropriate (deserving?) for rehabilitation services. It was sometime later, though my notes do not indicate when, that I developed the notion of detective work as a way to organize and further develop my understanding of rehabilitation and other human service work. I do not know why, although in retrospect I realize it probably made a difference that I teach courses in crime and juvenile delinquency and had recently read William Sanders's (1977) *Detective Work*. Other than that, I cannot say why I developed that framework. Certainly other metaphors could be used. Perhaps that is a creative, not explicit or knowable feature of doing sociological investigation. While social scientists attempt to demystify social life, I do not know that all of it can be demystified.

REASONABLE DOUBTS

Judges instruct juries that if they have any reasonable doubts as to the guilt of the accused, then their duty is to find the accused innocent. All social scientific investigations include limitations of the research and the findings. Those limitations may sometimes give rise to reasonable doubts. Typically they merely qualify the merit of the work to those who use the work.

I would have felt much more comfortable, though I am not sure my story would have changed significantly, if I could have observed the working of cases from beginning to conclusion. Due to my other responsibilities, such as teaching, I could not observe all day everyday for weeks and months. I saw bits and pieces. By putting those bits and pieces together, I developed a story of rehabilitation counselors and other human service professionals. Yet remember, detectives of all kinds put bits and pieces together, and their work days are mosaics of bits and pieces of activities.

Much of my understanding of rehabilitation work was based on talk about the work: counselors and other professionals talking to one another (about cases in a CDS for example) or to me (about their work in an interview or in a casual conversation). Of course, much of what counselors and other human service professionals do is done through talk (and writing). While approximately one-third of my typed notes (approximately 1000 pages) concerned observations of counselors' activities (independent of staffing), more direct observation of the interaction between counselors and clients might have been useful. And a fuller account of the work of rehabilitation detectives could have been achieved through an examination of the work done by state-level administrators and federal officials, both regional and national. From an investigation of such work, a better understanding of the larger organizational and national context of doing rehabilitation could be developed.

As in much field research, I observed one setting and one group of people within that setting. As noted in Chapter 1, the area office I observed was one of the most productive within a state that was nationally recognized as a leader in rehabilitation. Human service work, such as rehabilitation counseling, does vary according to the circumstances in which it is done (Galvin, 1974; Feinberg and McFarland, 1979). How it varies is, of course, important. However, to the extent that some of the counselors in the area office I observed had worked in other area offices, and to the extent that concerns about and problems of service stemming from an emphasis on goals is well documented throughout the nation, I suspect that the major points I have made regarding rehabilitation work have wide applicability. The similarities between rehabilitation work and the work of other human service professionals point to a wider applicability as well. As I noted in the Introduction, while many of the facts and figures will be forgotten soon (and may differ from setting to setting) the framework used to make sense of them can be used again and again. Through the metaphor of detective work, I have attempted to improve our understanding of rehabilitation and other human service work.

NOTES

1. Because there was turnover during my research, I calculated this figure based on those who were employed at the restart of my investigation in spring 1981. As new counselors appeared, I interviewed them.
2. See Johnson (1975: chap. 4) for a discussion of trust in field research.

References

Altheide, David L.
   1976   Creating Reality: How TV News Distorts Events. Beverly Hills, CA: Sage.
Atheide, David L. and John M. Johnson
   1980   Bureaucratic Propaganda. Boston: Allyn & Bacon.
Bell, Daniel
   1972   "Labor in the post-industrial society." Dissent 19: 163-189.
Berkowitz, Monroe, Valerie Englander, Jeffrey Rubin, and John D. Worral
   1975   An Evaluation of Policy-Related Rehabilitation Research. New York: Praeger.
Bitter, James A.
   1979   Introduction to Rehabilitation. St. Louis: C.V. Mosby.
Bitter, James A. and Joseph T. Kunce
   1979   "Counselors' perceptions of problems in delivery of services to the rural
           disabled disadvantaged." Rehabilitation Counseling Bulletin 15: 147-153
Blau, Peter M.
   1955   The Dynamics of Bureaucracy. Chicago: University of Chicago Press.
Blumer, Herbert
   1969   Symbolic Interactionism: Perspective and Method. Englewood Cliffs, NJ:
           Prentice-Hall.
Bogdan, Robert and Douglas Biklen
   1977   "Handicapism." Social Policy 7: 14-19.
Bogdan, Robert and Margaret Ksander
   1980   "Policy data as a social process: a qualitative approach to quantitative data."
           Human Organization 39: 302-309.
Bolton, Brian
   1978   "Methodological issues in the assessment of rehabilitation counselor per-
           formance." Rehabilitation Counseling Bulletin 21: 190-193.
Bowe, Frank
   1978   Handicapping America: Barriers to Disabled People. New York: Harper &
           Row.
   1980   Rehabilitating America: Toward Independence for Disabled and Elderly
           People. New York: Harper & Row.
Bowman, James T. and Leo A. Micek
   1973   "Rehabilitation service components and vocational outcome." Rehabilitation
           Counseling Bulletin 17: 101-109.
Bozarth, Jerold D. and Stanford E. Rubin
   1975   "Empirical observations of rehabilitation counselor performance and outcome:
           some implications." Rehabilitation Counseling Bulletin 19: 294-298.
Bozarth, Jerold D., Stanford E. Rubin, Conrad C. Krauft, Bill K. Richardson, and Brian
Bolton
   1974   "Client-counselor interaction, patterns of service, and client outcome: overview
           of project—conclusions and implications." Monograph 19. University of
           Arkansas, Arkansas Rehabilitation Research and Training Center.
Britten, Norman D.
   1981   "The art of vocational rehabilitation casework." Journal of Rehabilitation 47:
           71-80.
Buckholdt, David R. and Jaber F. Gubrium
   1979a Caretakers: Treating Emotionally Disturbed Children. Beverly Hills, CA:
           Sage.

1979b "Doing staffings." Human Organization 38: 255-264.

Colvin, Craig R.
1972 "The correctional institution and vocational rehabilitation," pp. 351-379 in John G. Cull and Richard E. Hardy (eds.) Vocational Rehabilitation: Profession and Process. Springfields, IL: Charles C Thomas.

Cooper, Paul and Reed Greenwood
1975 "Assessing undue delays in the vocational rehabilitation process," pp. 81-130 in Stanford E. Rubin (ed.) Studies on the Evaluation of State Vocational Rehabilitation Agency Programs: A Final Report. Fayetteville: University of Arkansas/Arkansas Rehabilitation Services, Arkansas Rehabilitation Research and Training Center.

Couch, Robert H.
1979 "Keeping score and looking good: the dilemma of certification in the private rehabilitation sector." Journal of Rehabilitation 45: 62-64.

Cox, Jennings G., Sean G. Connolly, and William J. Flynn
1981 "Managing the delivery of rehabilitation services," pp. 295-324 in Randall M. Parker and Carl E. Hansen (eds.) Rehabilitation Counseling Foundations-Consumers-Service Delivery. Boston: Allyn & Bacon.

Crisler, Jack R. and Joseph N. Edwards
1980 "Outcome measurement in the management control project." Journal of Rehabilitation 46: 31-35.

Crisler, Jack R., Timothy Fields, and Jean Pierson
1980 "Developing and implementing the management control project (MCP) in the Georgia DVR Agency." Journal of Rehabilitation 46: 52-57.

Crystal, Ralph M.
1981 "Counselors' perceptions of clients' needs." Rehabilitation Counseling Bulletin 24: 213-218.

Cull, John G. and Richard E. Hardy
1972 Vocational Rehabilitation: Profession and Process. Springfield, IL: Charles C Thomas.

Davis, Fred
1974 "Stories and sociology." Urban Life and Culture 3: 310-316.

DeJong, Gerben
1983 "Defining and implementing the independent living concept," pp. 4-27 in Nancy M. Crewe, Irving Kenneth Zola, and associates (eds.) Independent Living for Physically Disabled People. San Francisco: Jossey-Bass.

Di Michael, Salvatore
1969 "The current scene," pp. 5-28 in David Malikin and Herbert Rusalem (eds.) Vocational Rehabilitation of the Disabled: An Overview. New York: New York University Press.

Emener, William G.
1978 "An empirical investigation of rehabilitation counselor characteristics and client outcomes." Tallahassee: Florida State University.
1980 "Relationships among rehabilitation counselor characteristics and rehabilitation client outcomes." Rehabilitation Counseling Bulletin 23: 183-192.

Emener, William G. and Stanford E. Rubin
1980 "Rehabilitation counselor roles and functions and sources of role strain." Journal of Applied Rehabilitation Counseling 11: 57-69.

Emerson, Robert and Melvin Pollner
1978 "Policies and practices of psychiatric case selection." Sociology of Work and Occupations 5: 75-96.

Empey, LaMar T.
    1978   American Deliquency: Its Meaning and Construction. Homewood, IL:
            Dorsey.
Erickson, Frederick and Jeffery Shultz
    1982   The Counselor as Gatekeeper: Social Interaction in Interviews. New York:
            Academic.
Euler, Bryan
    1979   "Eligibility as a foundation for rehabilitation casework." Journal of Rehabili-
            tation 45: 52-55.
Farley, Roy C. and Stanford E. Rubin
    1980   "Rehabilitation counselor interaction style during the initial interview."
            Journal of Applied Rehabilitation Counseling 11: 44-45.
Feinberg, Lawrence B. and Fred R. McFarland
    1979   "Setting-based factors in rehabilitation counselor role variability." Journal of
            Applied Rehabilitation Counseling 10: 95-101.
Flannagan, Thomas
    1974   "What ever happened to placement?" Vocational Guidance Quarterly 22:
            209-213.
Freidson, Eliot
    1975   Doctoring Together: A Study of Professional Control. New York: Elsevier.
Galvin, Donald E.
    1974   "Program evaluation in Michigan VR service." Social and Rehabilitation
            Record 1: 28-31.
General Accounting Office (GAO)
    1973   Effectiveness of Vocational Rehabilitation in Helping the Handicapped.
            Report to the Congress. Washington, DC: Author.
    1977   Controls over Vocational Rehabilitation Training Services Need Improvement.
            Report to the Congress. Washington, DC: Author.
    1978   Third Party Funding Agreements: No Longer Appropriate for Serving the
            Handicapped Through the Vocational Rehabilitation Program. Report to the
            Congress. Washington, DC: Author.
    1982   Improved Administration of the Vocational Rehabilitation Program Would
            Provide More Effective Utilization of Program Funds. Washington, DC:
            Author.
Gartner, Alan
    1977   "Consumers in the Services Society." Social Policy 8: 2-8.
Gartner, Alan, Colin Greer, and Frank Riessman (eds.)
    1979   Consumer Education in the Human Services. New York: Pergamon.
Gell, Frank
    1969   The Black Badge: Confessions of a Caseworker. New York: Harper & Row.
Gibbs, Jack P. and Maynard L. Erickson
    1979   "Conceptions of criminal and deliquent acts." Deviant Behavior 1: 71-100.
Gilsinan, James, F.
    1982   Doing Justice: How the System Works—As Seen by the Participants.
            Englewood Cliffs, NJ: Prentice-Hall.
Goffman, Erving
    1952   "On cooling the mark out: some aspects of adaptation to failure." Psychiatry
            15: 451-463.

Goldin, George J.
 1966 "Some rehabilitation counselor attitudes toward their professional role." Rehabilitation Literature 27: 360-364.
Growick, Bruce S. and Dean Stueland
 1979 "The relationship between differential service patterns and change in weekly earnings for three disability groups." Rehabilitation Counseling Bulletin 22: 431-435.
Gubrium, Jaber F.
 1980a "Doing care plans in patient conferences." Social Science and Medicine 14A: 659-667.
 1980b "Patient exclusion in geriatric staffings." Sociological Quarterly 21: 335-347.
Gubrium, Jaber F. and David R. Buckholdt
 1979 "Production of hard data in human service institutions." Pacific Sociological Review 22: 115-136.
 1982 Describing Care: Image and Practice in Rehabilitation. Cambridge, MA: Oelgeschlager, Gunn, & Hain.
Gusfield, Joseph
 1976 "The literary rhetoric of science: comedy and pathos in drinking driver research." American Sociological Review 41: 16-34.
Guthrie, Joann L., Kerry Crist, Deborah A. Sienicki, and Richard T. Walls
 1981 "Homemaker rehabilitation in the age of accountability." Rehabilitation Literature 42: 90-94.
Hasenfeld, Yeheskel
 1972 "People processing organizations: an exchange approach." American Sociological Review 37: 256-263.
 1980 "Review: people processing." Journal of Social Service Research 3: 429-430.
Hasenfeld, Yeheskel and Richard A. English
 1974a (eds.) Human Service Organizations: A Book of Readings. Ann Arbor: University of Michigan Press.
 1974b "Human service organizations: a conceptual overview," pp. 1-32 in Yeheskel Hansenfeld and Richard A. English (eds.) Human Service Organizations: A Book of Readings. Ann Arbor: University of Michigan Press.
Haug, Marie R. and Marvin B. Sussman
 1968 "Professionalism and the public." Sociological Inquiry 39: 57-64.
Haug, Marie R., Marvin B. Sussman, and Kathleen Staruch
 1974 "The public views rehabilitation and human service careers." Working Paper 4, Rehabilitation Occupations for the Disadvantaged. and Advantaged. Case Western Reserve University.
Higgins, Paul C.
 1980 Outsiders in a Hearing World: A Sociology of Deafness. Beverly Hills, CA: Sage.
Higgins, Paul C. and Richard R. Butler
 1982 Understanding Deviance. New York: McGraw-Hill.
Huber, Milton J.
 1977 "26 million low-income consumers." Social Policy 8: 24-29.
Illich, Ivan
 1971 Deschooling Society. New York: Harper & Row.
 1975 Medical Nemesis: The Expropriation of Health. London: Calder & Boyars.

Illich, Ivan, Irving Kenneth Zola, John McKnight, Jonathan Caplan and Harley Shaiken
    1977   Disabling Professions. London: Marion Boyars.
Johnson, John M.
    1975   Doing Field Research. New York: Free Press.
Johnston, L. T.
    1975   "The counselor: as he really is." Journal of Rehabilitation 23: 9-10.
Ju, Jean Jiemean
    1982   "Counselor variables and rehabilitation outcomes: a literature overview."
            Journal of Applied Rehabilitation Counseling 13: 28-43.
Klein, Michael A., John D. Swisher, Ross Lynch, and Clark Krewson
    1982   "The rehabilitation counselor and the medical consultant." Rehabilitation
            Counseling Bulletin 25: 239-241.
Krause, Elliott A.
    1965   "Structured Strain in a marginal profession: rehabilitation counseling."
            Journal of Health and Human Behavior 6: 55-62.
Kunce, Joseph T., Douglas E. Miller and Corrine S. Cope
    1974   "Macro data analysis and rehabilitation program evaluation." Rehabilitation
            Counseling Bulletin 17: 132-140.
Lang, Claire Larracey
    1981   "Good cases-bad cases." Urban Life 10: 289-309.
Lassiter, Robert A.
    1972   "History of the rehabilitation movement in America," pp. 5-58 in John G. Cull
            and Richard E. Hardy (eds.) Vocational Rehabilitation: Profession and
            Process. Springfield, IL: Charles C Thomas.
Leary, Paul A. and M. S. Tseng
    1974   "Violence to the spirit of independence." Journal of Rehabilitation 42: 27-28,
            47-48.
Link, Bruce
    1982   "Mental patient status, work, and income: an examination of the effects of a
            psychiatric label." American Sociological Review 47: 202-215.
Lipsky, Michael
    1976   "Toward a theory of street-level bureaucracy," pp. 196-213 in Willis D. Hawley
            and Michael Lipsky (eds.) Theoretical Perspectives on Urban Politics.
            Englewood Cliffs, NJ: Prentice-Hall.
    1980   Street-Level Bureaucracy: Dilemmas of the Individual in Public Services. New
            York: Russell Sage.
Lofquist, Lloyd
    1969   "Selected techniques of counseling," pp. 217-236 in David Malikin and Herbert
            Rusalem (eds.) Vocational Rehabilitation of the Disabled: An Overview. New
            York: New York University Press.
Lundman, Richard J., Richard E. Sykes, and John P. Clark
    1978   "Police control of juveniles: a replication." Journal of Research in Crime and
            Delinquency 15: 74-91.
McCleary, Richard
    1978   Dangerous Men: The Sociology of Parole. Beverly Hills, CA: Sage.
McCleary, Richard, Barbara C. Nienstedt, and James M. Erven
    1982   "Uniform crime reports as organizational outcomes: three time series experi-
            ments." Social Problems 29: 361-372.

McDaniel, Randall S.
   1979   "Southeast rehabilitation counselors' views of vocational evaluation services."
           Journal of Applied Rehabilitation Counseling 9: 178-183.
McGowan, John
   1969   "Referral, evaluation, treatment," pp. 111-128 in David Malikin and Herbert
           Rusalem (eds.) Vocational Rehabilitation of the Disabled: An Overview. New
           York: New York University Press.
McKinlay, John B.
   1978   "The limits of human services." Social Policy 8: 29-34.
Malikin, David and Herbert Rusalem (eds.)
   1969   Vocational Rehabilitation of the Disabled: An Overview. New York: New York
           University Press.
Manning, Peter K.
   1974   "Police lying." Urban Life and Culture 3: 283-306.
Manus, Gerald I.
   1975   "Is your language disabling?" Journal of Rehabilitation 41: 35.
Mayer, John E. and Aaron Rosenblatt
   1975   "Encounters with danger: social workers in the ghetto." Sociology of Work and
           Occupations 2: 227-245.
Miller, Gale
   1983   "Holding clients accountable: the micro-politics of trouble in a work incentive
           program." Social Problems 31: 129-151.
Morris, Norval and Gordon Hawkins
   1970   The Honest Politician's Guide to Crime Control. Chicago: University of
           Chicago Press.
Murphy, Stephen T. and Alex Ursprung
   1983   "The politics of vocational evaluation: a qualitative study." Rehabilitation
           Literature 44: 1-12, 18.
Muthard, John
   1969   "The status of the profession," pp. 275-305 in David Malikin and Herbert
           Rusalem (eds.) Vocational Rehabilitation of the Disabled: An Overview. New
           York: New York University Press.
Muthard, John E. and Paul R. Salomone
   1969   "The roles and functions of rehabilitation counselors." Rehabilitation Counsel-
           ing Bulletin 13: 81-168.
Nagi, Saad Z.
   1974   "Gate-keeping decisions in service organizations: when validity fails." Human
           Organization 33: 47-58.
Obermann, C. Esco
   1965   A History of Vocational Rehabilitation in America. Minneapolis: T.S.
           Denison.
Olshansky, Simon
   1976   "Counseling, state vocational rehabilitation agencies, and related matters."
           Rehabilitation Literature 37: 263-267, 288.
   1981   "Some responses of vocational rehabilitation counselors to job placement."
           Rehabilitation Literature 42: 23-25.
Peyrot, Mark
   1982   "Caseload management: choosing suitable clients in a community health clinic
           agency." Social Problems 30: 157-167.

Pinkerton, Susan S. and Susan B. Nelson
   1978   "Counselor variables influencing rehabilitation outcome of persons with
          cancer." Rehabilitation Counseling Bulletin 22: 253-260.
President's Commission on Law Enforcement and Administration of Justice
   1967   Task Force Report: Juvenile Delinquency and Youth Crime. Washington, DC:
          Government Printing Office.
Prottas, Jeffrey Manditch
   1979   People-Processing: The Street-Level Bureaucrat in Public Service Bureau-
          cracies. Lexington, MA: D.C. Heath.
Reagles, Kenneth W., George N. Wright, and Alfred J. Butler
   1971   "Rehabilitation gain: relationship with client characteristics and and counselor
          intervention." Journal of Counseling Psychology 18: 490-495.
Rehabilitation Services Administration (RSA)
   1981   Annual Report of the Rehabilitation Services Administration to the President
          and the Congress on Federal Activities Related to the Administration of the
          Rehabilitation Act of 1973, as Amended. Fiscal Year 1981. Washington, DC:
          U.S. Department of Education, Office of Special Education and Rehabilitative
          Services.
   1982a Caseload Statistics, State Vocational Rehabilitation Agencies, Fiscal Year
          1981. Washington, DC: U.S. Department of Education, Office of Special
          Education and Rehabilitative Services.
   1982b Characteristics of Persons Rehabilitated in Fiscal Year 1980. Washington, DC:
          U.S. Department of Education, Office of Special Education and Rehabilitative
          Services.
   1983   Caseload Statistics, State Vocational Rehabilitation Agencies, Fiscal Year
          1982. Washington, DC: U.S. Department of Education, Office of Special
          Education and Rehabilitative Services.
   1984   Caseload Statistics, State Vocational Rehabilitation Agencies, Fiscal Year
          1983. Washington, DC: U.S. Department of Education, Office of Education
          and Rehabilitative Services.
Reiman, Jeffrey H.
   1984   The Rich Get Richer and the Poor Get Prison: Ideology, Class and Criminal
          Justice. New York: John Wiley.
Rein, Mildred
   1980   "Fact and function in human service organizations." Sociology and Social
          Research 65: 78-93.
Roth, Juluis A.
   1972   "Some contingencies of the moral evaluation and control of clientele: the case
          of the hospital emergency service." American Journal of Sociology 77: 839-856.
Rubin, Stanford E.
   1975   (ed.) Studies on the Evaluation of State Vocational Rehabilitation Agency
          Programs: A Final Report. Fayetteville: University of Arkansas/Arkansas
          Rehabilitation Services, Arkansas Rehabilitation Research and Training
          Center.
   1977   "A national rehabilitation program evaluation research and training effort:
          some results and implications." Journal of Rehabilitation 43: 28-31.
Rubin, Stanford E. and Paul G. Cooper
   1977   "A placement suitability measure for assessing rehabilitation service units."
          Rehabilitation Counseling Bulletin 21: 23-29.
Rubin, Stanford E. and William G. Emener
   1979   "Recent rehabilitation counselor role changes and role strain—a pilot investiga-
          tion." Journal of Applied Rehabilitation Counseling 10: 142-147.

Salomone, Paul R.
  1970   "Disability: a re-conceptualization." Journal of Rehabilitation 36: 14-17.
  1972   "Client motivation and rehabilitation counseling outcome." Rehabilitation Counseling Bulletin 16: 11-20.
Salomone, Paul R. and William M. Usdane
  1977   "Client-centered placement revisited: a dialogue on placement philosophy." Rehabilitation Counseling Bulletin 21: 85-91, 176.
Sanders, William B.
  1976   The Sociologist as Detective: An Introduction to Research Methods. New York: Praeger.
  1977   Detective Work: A Study of Criminal Investigations. New York: Free Press.
  1980   Rape and Woman's Identity. Beverly Hills, CA: Sage.
Singer, Benjamin D.
  1980   "Crazy systems." Social Policy 11: 46-54.
Sinick, Daniel,
  1969   "Training, job placement, follow-up," pp. 129-154 in David Malikin and Herbert Rusalem (eds.) Vocational Rehabilitation of the Disabled: An Overview. New York: New York University Press.
Skolnick, Jerome H.
  1966   Justice Without Trial. New York: John Wiley.
Skolnick, Jerome H. and Richard Woodworth
  1967   "Bureaucracy, information, and social control: a study of a morals detail," pp. 99-136 in David J. Bordua (ed.) The Police: Six Sociological Essays. New York: John Wiley.
Smits, Stanley J. and James G. Ledbetter
  1979   "The practice of rehabilitation counseling within the administrative structure of the state-federal program." Journal of Applied Rehabilitation Counseling 10: 78-84.
Stewart, Robert L. and Charles W. Tucker
  1983   "Research for what? Notes on Mead's pragmatic theory of truth." (mimeo)
Sudnow, David
  1965   "Normal crimes: sociological features of the penal code in a public defender office." Social Problems 12: 255-276.
Sussman, Marvin B.
  1972   "A policy perspective on the United States rehabilitation system." Journal of Health and Social Behavior 13: 152-161.
Sussman, Marvin B. and Marie R. Haug
  1970   "From student to practitioner: professionalization and deprofessionalization in rehabilitation counseling." Working Paper No. 7. Case Western Reserve University.
Sussman, Marvin B., Marie R. Haug, and Vivian Joynes
  1969   "Rehabilitation within a climate of change," in Professions Project Research Dissemination and Utilization Conference. Cleveland: Case Western Reserve University.
Switzer, Mary
  1969   "Legislative contributions," pp. 39-52 in David Malikin and Herbert Rusalem (eds.) Vocational Rehabilitation of the Disabled: An Overview. New York: New York University Press.

Thomas, Kenneth R., Jean O. Britton, and Shlomo P. Kravetz
    1974   "Vocational rehabilitation counselors view the Judeo-Christian work ethic."
            Rehabilitation Counseling Bulletin 18: 105-111.
Tseng, M. S. and W. Dennis Zarega
    1976   "The intake, process, and outcome performance of vocational rehabilitation in
            the field." Rehabilitation Literature 37: 343-346.
U.S. Department of Justice
    1981   Criminal Victimization in the United States, 1979. Washington, DC: Bureau of
            Justice Statistics.
Usdane, William M. and Paul R. Salomone
    1977   "Reconceptualization of the placement process: a dialogue." Rehabilitation
            Counseling Bulletin 21: 92-102.
Vandergroot, David
    1981   "Placement and career development counseling in rehabilitation," pp. 261-293
            in Randall M. Parker and Carl E. Hansen (eds.) Rehabilitation Counseling:
            Foundations-Consumers-Service Delivery. Boston: Allyn & Bacon.
Vandergroot, David and James Engelkes
    1980   "The relationship of selected rehabilitation counseling variables with job-
            seeking behaviors." Rehabilitation Counseling Bulletin 24: 173-177.
Vernon, McCay, Phillip Bussey, and Deborah S. Day.
    1979   "The 'closure system' and accountability in vocational rehabilitation." Journal
            of Rehabilitation 45: 45-47.
Waegel, William B.
    1981   "Case routinization in investigative police work." Social Problems 28: 263-275.
Walls, Richard T. and Joseph B. Moriarity
    1977   "The caseload profile: an alternative to weighted closure." Rehabilitation
            Literature 38: 285-291.
Warren, Carol A.B.
    1980   "Data presentation and the audience: responses, ethics, and effects." Urban
            Life 9: 282-308.
Warren, Sol L.
    1959   "The rehabilitation counselor today: what, where, and why." Journal of
            Rehabilitation 25: 7-9.
Weatherly, Richard A.
    1979   Reforming Special Education: Policy Implementation from State Level to
            Street Level. Cambridge: MIT Press.
Whitehouse, Frederick A.
    1975   "Rehabilitation clinician." Journal of Rehabilitation 41: 24-26.
Willey, Douglas A.
    1979   "Caseload management for the vocational rehabilitation counselor in a state
            agency." Journal of Applied Rehabilitation Counseling 9: 152-158.
Williams, J. Allen, Jr., and Agnes M. Edwards
    1971   "Rehabilitation and the black community." Journal of Rehabilitation 37:
            43-46.
Worrall, John D. and David Vandergroot
    1980   "Indicators fo nonsuccess for early vocational rehabilitation intervention."
            Rehabilitation Counseling Bulletin 23: 282-290.
    1982   "Additional indicators of nonsuccess: a follow-up report." Rehabilitation
            Counseling Bulletin 26: 88-93.

Wright, George Nelson
1980   Total Rehabilitation. Boston: Little, Brown.
York, Phyllis, David York, and Ted Wachtel
1982   Toughlove. Garden City, NY: Doubleday.
Zadny, Jerry J. and Leslie F. James
1976   "Another view of placement: state of the art 1976." Studies in Placement Monograph No. 1. Portland State University, Regional Rehabilitation Research Institute.
1977a "A review of research on job placement." Rehabilitation Counseling Bulletin 21: 151-158.
1977b "Time spent on placement." Rehabilitation Counseling Bulletin 21: 31-35.
1978   "A survey of job-search patterns among state vocational rehabilitation clients." Rehabilitation Counseling Bulletin 22: 60-65.
1979a "Job placement in state vocational rehabilitation agencies: a survey technique." Rehabilitation Counseling Bulletin 22: 361-379.
1979b "The problem with placement." Rehabilitation Counseling Bulletin 22: 439-442.
Zimmerman, Don H.
1966   "Paper work and people work: a study of a public assistance agency." Doctoral dissertation, University of California, Los Angeles.

About the Author

Paul C. Higgins is an Associate Professor of Sociology who researches and writes in the areas of deviance and disability. Among his books are *Outsiders in a Hearing World* and *Understanding Deviance* (with Richard Butler).